PRAISE FOR *SURPRISED BY JOY*

'*Surprised by Joy* isn't a breath of fresh air—it's a fierce, passionate, tender sirocco blowing straight from the beating heart of Africa. It tells the story of one man's extraordinary journey from suburban Dublin to the African bush, and his spiritual quest for fulfilment. Michael Meegan practises what so many only preach: how to show compassion, feel love, give hope. This book blasts throu̶ ̶̶̶̶̶̶̶̶̶̶ions of poverty and suffering an̶ ̶̶̶̶̶̶̶̶̶̶̶̶̶̶̶̶̶elp itself. Both hum ̶̶̶̶̶̶̶̶̶̶̶̶̶̶̶̶̶̶̶̶you wondering who ̶̶̶̶̶̶̶̶̶̶̶̶̶̶̶̶̶̶̶̶ose who have nothi̶ ̶̶̶̶̶̶̶̶̶̶̶̶̶̶̶̶̶̶elp.' - Lise Hand, *The ̶̶̶̶̶̶̶̶̶̶̶̶̶*

'There are many wounds on the face of this earth. Our world is starved of love. It longs to be held and healed. Mike Meegan has heard this call and embraced it without prejudice. In reaching out to those who are most vulnerable, he has touched a profound spiritual truth—that service to another is an expression of the search for a unifying love, and not just a desire for social change.' - Liam Lawton, *Composer*

'Mike Meegan's life story is testament to the authenticity of his humanity. This is a story of love, spirituality and hard humanitarian graft in the poor world. In these pages we are reintroduced to the sacred within all of us and to the awesome life-altering power of grace. The book is also an important scholarly work on the effectiveness of Aid to the global poor grounded on medical-based research.' - Liz O'Donnell, *T.D.*

Surprised By Joy

Out of the Darkness, Light;
A Story of Hope in the Midst of Tragedy

by Michael Meegan

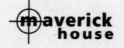

Published by Maverick House Publishers.

Maverick House, Main Street, Dunshaughlin, Co. Meath, Ireland.
Maverick House SE Asia, 440 Sukhumvit Road, Washington Square,
Klongton, Klongtoey, Bangkok 10110, Thailand.

info@maverickhouse.com
http://www.maverickhouse.com

ISBN: 1-905379-05-6
978-1-905379-05-7

5 4 3 2 1

The paper used in this book comes from wood pulp of managed
forests. For every tree felled at least one tree is planted, thereby
renewing natural resources.

Printed by Mackays of Chatham Ltd.

A CIP catalogue record for this book is available from the British
Library.

DEDICATION

In life we are blessed with many wonderful gifts. The most amazing of these are the people who come into our lives and just decide for no reason at all to love us. These are the people who accept us completely, just as we are. There is nothing more healing or completing than the rare friends who know our inner selves. They are the soul bonds, the friends who rejoice with us, hold our hand as we explore together.

Sharon is such a light in my life. She is always celebrating, sharing, reaching out to me. She is that rare fire that brings renewal and laughter, joy and meaning. Sharon, this is for you.

ACKNOWLEDGEMENTS

We can only live our dreams if we believe in ourselves. It is easy to believe in the impossible when your life is full of those who dream with you.

To everyone who has held my hand, everyone who has embraced me, everyone who has rejoiced with me, my kiss.

To the friends who have loved me and filled me with their magic, you have my heart.

To those who have shared their spirit and their light, touched my life and enriched it with their beauty, my embrace.

To those who have brought me into the sanctuary of their hearts and accepted me in all my frailty, my breath is yours.

To those who walk at my side and celebrate this adventure, you fill my life so much.

To those awake, amazed, and full of wonder in the mystery, it is unfolding.

For the endless grace, kindness, acts of love, I leave it to One greater than I to thank you, for in all things I am astonished and each moment increasingly surprised by joy.

FOREWORD

In the summer of 2005 I was preparing for a trip to Africa to record a series of interviews for my *HARDtalk* programme on BBC TV. All the talk in London that June was of Bono and Geldof; their *Live8* extravaganza and Tony Blair's ambition to put global poverty at the top of the agenda at the forthcoming G8 summit in Gleneagles.

I had already fixed a series of interviews with prime ministers, opposition leaders and top diplomats—the typical Big Men of Africa—but something told me I needed more: a different perspective, a fresh voice.

An American journalist, Jennifer Glass, whom I'd known as a brave and tenacious colleague in Baghdad but who had previously spent years working in Nairobi, gave me a steer for which I will forever be grateful.

'Try a guy called Michael Meegan,' she said. 'He's doing unbelievable work in the Kenyan bush, and I guarantee he'll give you an interview you'll never forget.'

Three weeks later my crew and I were rattling down a dirt road into the shimmering heat of the Rift Valley. But as we headed towards Meegan's remote clinic in the desiccated Maasai country my mood was gloomy.

In the previous days I'd had encounters that confirmed my worst fears about the crisis in African governance. In Addis Ababa, Ethiopian Prime Minister Meles Zenawi—anointed by Tony Blair as the very model of progressive African leadership-had defended his security forces' suppression of opposition protests with lethal gunfire. 'A necessary defence against criminals' he called it, with more than a trace of menace. Ethiopia, one of the poorest countries on earth, was, it seemed, in danger of sliding into political chaos.

In Nairobi I'd found a Kenyan Government and opposition trading accusations about rampant corruption. The official charged with investigating allegations of kickbacks, money laundering and ministerial graft had quit, claiming intimidation. Ordinary Kenyans, facing a savage drought across much of the country, appeared to have little, if any, expectation of honesty or competence from their rulers.

And so I brought to my encounter with this Irish/English doctor, of whom I knew very little, a whole bagful of preconceptions. Another do-gooder I thought; a white outsider with a bleeding heart, fuelled by anger and guilt. An aid peddlar engaged in an ultimately futile attempt to overcome the failings of Western and African political leadership.

And then I actually met Michael Meegan.

He was youthful and wiry. If he was burdened with the woes of the world's poorest people, it didn't show. And he was, from the very first moment, a compelling, barely-pausing, continent-hopping teller of stories. He talked as if energised by the African sun itself.

Our conversation didn't develop in the way I had anticipated. I'd expected anger, cynicism and frustration. What I found was hope, wonder and yes, even joy. I asked questions about hopelessness and despair. I got answers about love and kindness.

Michael Meegan is no idle dreamer. I've seen the work he does; the local staff he's helped to train. His work on disease control has helped countless thousands, not just in Africa but across the world. But what sets him apart is how he's chosen to make his journey. With his heart open. With a conviction that love is the greatest healer of all. For those of us infected with cynicism, sometimes weary of a broken world, Meegan's life offers more than inspiration. It points us towards a cure.

– Stephen Sackur, *HARDtalk*, BBC Television.

INTRODUCTION

I met Mike Meegan not long after he died. He wasn't the first person I met who had died, either. The first person was a woman who had waited until the bank holiday weekend when her flatmates were away, and had taken a lethal overdose of medication. All weekend she lay on the floor in a coma, so that by the time her flatmates returned the parts of her body she had been lying on were rotting from lack of blood. She was alive, though, and she recovered in hospital. I watched her as she took part in the routine life of the psychiatric unit I was working in. She watched everything with a curious eye, looking at a cup of coffee she shouldn't have been alive to drink, a newspaper whose news should have happened after her death, whose news might even have included her death. No-one believed there was a significant risk that she would make another attempt, at least not right away. The detachment of her gaze was startling. Everything was curious, and nothing really mattered, because she had survived her own death and was seeing a life that came after it.

I didn't realise it at first, but neither, I think, did Mike. But he had died just before I met him, and was living the life that comes after death. It happened just as he had always thought it would. It was down near the Tanzanian border in a place where there aren't any things on the map and, when you look, the map is just about right. Mike was down there when he suddenly fell very seriously ill. Too ill to think about trying to drive across the bush and back to the road. There was no other driver with him, just some Maasai, so there he stayed, being cared for the Maasai, as his temperature soared. His legs swelled up grotesquely, he became delirious, he went blind. But something in him knew that this was the time. He wasn't going to get better. And this didn't matter. He was here, under the wide African sky he loved, surrounded by the sounds of Maasai speaking quietly, being tended lovingly by those he had worked with and given his life to. He had come to Africa to give his life in the service of those who needed it, he had followed Jesus' challenge, he had given it all away and for his reward he was ending his life in a place that seemed the sweetest spot on earth, among people who are endlessly wonderful.

I know the place, the people, all this is true. There is great peace out there. So Mike felt his life ebb without fear or regrets. Certainly, there was so much left undone, but the important thing was that he had given his life for what he believed in. Gradually, he lost consciousness. It was finished.

Of course, it wasn't. Gradually, he got better. It was a long time before he was able to drive, and for the first few years I knew him, Mike would have to get his legs massaged for half an hour every morning before he was able to walk. Even at that, he staggered around stiffly for the first half of the day. No-one ever knew what the disease was. So I missed the first Mike, the Mike who had a simple mission and who waited, wracked with fever, like a ripe apple, waiting for God to pluck him For His Time Had Come.

The Mike I met was an unsettled, unsettling person. There are images of the first Mike, a gaunt, unshaven young man who seemed always to be holding an emaciated child when anyone photographed him (did he ever put them down, I wondered). He had written a book called *All Shall Be Well*, which seemed to me like the most blatant self-deception possible. Of course All Shall Not Be Well unless we get to work, I thought, and even then we stand to get very little done. It sounded to me like the sort of wishful thinking you could do if you didn't notice that All Was Not Well with the emaciated child in your arms.

How could anyone who found a child like this say something like *All Shall Be Well?* What's the point, I thought—the child may soon not be able to hear you. It will be dead. I have children. Any parent can imagine their little ones, trying to hold on to someone, dying. Any parent would tear their heart out sooner than see one of their children die like this. In a world where small children die like this, all is not well. And that's hard to understand.

I taught in Milltown Institute of Theology and Philosophy—in fact, I just missed teaching Mike. I was on the philosophy faculty. Between philosophers and theologians, there was no telling what sort of coffee break conversation you would have. One Friday the staff room was unusually merry. One of the other lecturers told me the story. The previous night there had been a meeting of prominent members of the Catholic laity and some of the theologians had been invited. Over refreshments afterwards, one wealthy and successful man was complaining loudly. 'Why can't ordinary people see,' he asked, 'that whatever happens is God's will and is all for the best?'

'I don't know,' said the theologian. 'I reckon that believing in God is more like being married to the moors murderer. When He comes home in the evening, you give Him His tea. But you don't ever ask Him what He did today.'

It's hard to start life in your late thirties. And very strange to watch. I spent a lot of time with Mike, talking, arguing (it's what we Irish do best), drinking beer, walking around the bush, sitting in the sauna at the gym. We're both anecdotal people, Mike and I. But over the years, I've noticed a change in both of us. In Mike's case, the stories have got less simple and obvious. The first Mike wrote about the simple goodness of people, of a shepherd boy who gave the only piece of clothing he had to a little refugee whose language he couldn't even speak. Now I knew the full story—the shepherd boy wasn't just a saint, he was also a crook, who was fired for stealing and selling ICROSS goats. And that's what appealed to me about him.

We don't want to know that there are people on the face of the earth who are far more wonderful than we are. We want to know that we, too, are capable of better things. That even crooks can be kind. The present Mike is more difficult to read precisely because the moral isn't always obvious anymore. The story or stories chase one another through the pages, characters turn up, have adventures, vanish again, and the moral is less clear than ever. But the exhilaration is all the more obvious. Sarune, of whom Mike speaks a lot, is a remarkable person who speaks to the living and dead alike. He sometimes turns up in dreams. He arrived in one of mine, once. In my dream, we were looking out over the bush and I saw some Maasai grandmothers walking in the distance.

I asked Sarune how the Maasai could walk such vast distances—Maasai think nothing of setting out to pay a call on someone who lives four day's walk away. Sarune smiled and said that you didn't think about the distance, or, if maybe if you did think about it, you thought that you were closer to your destination than the last time you thought about it. And in my dream I got very irritated by this sort of pocket Buddha answer, and I said angrily, 'But what if your journey has no destination?'

Sarune simply smiled and said, 'Then you are simply out for a walk.'

Mike is a person out on a walk. A good place to be.

– Dr Ronan Conroy, Department of Tropical Medicine, Royal College of Surgeons, Ireland.

PROLOGUE

We have forgotten the secrets of happiness and have lost the art of wonder. Our world is in pain, and the gap between nations grows. The problems seem overwhelming.

Recently, I was interviewed by Stephen Sackur on BBC's *HARDtalk*. In that interview, I was asked many tough questions, to which there are no easy answers. Stephen asked me about poverty, corruption, suffering and disease. He asked me why I do what I do and why I wasn't angry.

The huge response to this interview included an invitation from Maverick House Publishers to write this book, with all proceeds going to charity. It is the first of two books. It is a more complete reflection on the critical questions raised in the initial BBC interview, and an account of my life, my influences and the development of my beliefs and ideas over time, in an attempt to explain how I came to do what I do and be who I am today.

In a departure from their normal subject matter, they wanted to publish a book that would tackle a new way of looking at international aid, and agreed to cover the costs. Unlike many other works produced for charity, this book, thanks to their generosity, will see the proceeds of every sale donated to ICROSS.

This book tries to answer the questions I am asked all the time. People ask me how all of this came about. They ask me why I am so happy, why I am not frustrated or tired, why I don't become burnt out with the endless suffering and extreme poverty we work amongst.

This autobiographical reflection attempts to answer some of these questions. Not every question, however, needs an answer, and not every challenge has a solution. Our world has become confined in limited ways of reasoning. We often think in boxes. We want people to fit into our mental constructs of how things should be. A lot of people want you to fit into the categories and boxes they create. They form very rigid ideas of what being spiritual means. They have expectations of how you should behave and how you should conform. I have always believed that in being ourselves we should do what is within us and live our own dreams, never relying on how other people define us.

This book is above all about living your own mystery and tasting life, believing in your heart. We sometimes let fear get in the way of our dreams and we conform because it is safe and familiar. Each of us is many selves, many parts, many intelligences, as this story of my life shows.

If we learn to explore life using all of our energies we will celebrate every moment in a new and original way. We will see everything with amazement and we will be awoken—we will become the energy and love we want in the world.

Surprised by Joy is in part recollections of a journey full of ordinary experiences made extraordinary. It's about looking at life in a different way and sharing some of the lessons and knowledge I have learnt and gathered along the way.

Each of us has moments of doubt and frailty. All of us share the need to be cherished and hugged, and every one of us needs kindness and fulfilment. We all have dreams and hopes.

In sharing my own little journey, I hope that you will find within it something that can touch your heart. In my tears I hope you sense what I felt, and in my wonder I hope we share the same delight.

Of course there is tragedy, of course there is mindless cruelty. The bloodiness of man and the madness of war destroys so much hope. The suicides of lost and broken men, the tears of children and fears of starving mothers are here and now. Yes, there is apathy and corruption, and of course there is greed and oppression. Yet despite all of these things and more, regardless of suffering, there is also something else. I am increasingly amazed that despite all the badness in the world, there is so much love. There is so much raw goodness, pure kindness and compassion.

It is what exists despite the brokenness of humanity, its bizarre appetite for unkindness and perverse politics that make this story worth sharing. Having lived many lives and travelled many roads, the time is now right for me to illuminate some of the shadows, and try to share the joy I have been blessed with.

So many people ask me all the time if I ever feel overwhelmed in Africa. The answer is that of course I feel overwhelmed. I am overwhelmed by the happiness; the laughter; the fun and joy; the tranquility; the power and energy.

Deeper than these things is the realisation that we create happiness. It lives within this moment; in this miracle of now. The gift we give ourselves is this presence. We can take over our own lives. This story is not really about my being in Africa or about adventures. It is about being in ourselves and seeing the world through different eyes, with a new heart.

This reflection is about a very ordinary person with the same tastes and interests as most people. I dance and ski, love parties, enjoy restaurants and holidays with friends. Perhaps it is the things we have in common that make our different experiences meaningful. All of our lives somehow reflect the mystery and miracle of each other. All our experiences enrich each other. I share my life story with the awareness that it can never reflect the reality of experience. Our words are always shadows, dim shadows that vaguely hint at what we truly feel. It is only with our hearts that we truly speak, and only with each moment of our lives that we can give meaning to the absurdity and chaos of a torn world.

I share some of the lessons I have learnt in the hope that they might in some way be of value to others. This is a simple journey, a story of a child trying to find his way home, and of a pilgrim who has seen unimaginable suffering and sorrow, but also tremendous joy. There are simple paths that can bring us awesome joy and incredible pleasure. The secrets of joy are surprisingly simple and the way of compassion is a journey we become together. Perhaps the journey is not to practise acts of compassion but for us to become compassion itself.

Like all journeys, mine began in curiosity—excited and in awe of this fragile gift called life.

CHAPTER ONE

'Remember it is never your picture that is too big; sometimes the paper you are given might be too small, but whatever you do, make it as big as you want. Don't stop because of the paper.'
- *My old primary school teacher, Sr Oliver*

If your awakening is full of joy, so too shall be your day. If you are awake in your dawn, you shall see miracles unfold before you. That is an idea I live by.

I had a wonderful childhood, spent in amazement and discovery. I had such a great time that I decided to spend the rest of my life exploring. I decided to always love that child within me. The thing about curiosity is that the more doors you open, the more things there are to fill you with delight.

As a child growing up in Lancashire, I lived in Freshfield. It was an old cosy village like the ones in the Agatha Christie films. Mrs Cotgrieve ran the greengrocer's and no one ever remembered seeing a policeman. The police station was in Formby, and so was the toy shop. There was a great pine forest with a red squirrel colony and I used to go and feed them, and thought that everywhere must smell of flowers and plants. We never had television and never missed it, but we did have a childhood filled with innocence and wonder. It was a simple, unhurried world, and left an indelible impression upon my world view that something this great was worth sharing.

We moved around a lot, between England and Ireland, where my granny lived, and this gave me a great sense of a world outside of my family, my house, my neighbourhood.

My mother was a teacher and was loving and gentle. She had an understanding of what it meant to view the world as a child and was quite happy to let us discover it in our own way and at our own pace. Mum taught art and never looked at anything in a conventional way. She always saw shades and shadows, profusions of colours and subtleties of light. There was a tenderness in her art, and another pleasure for her was gardening. Mum never saw a cloud bringing rain; only one that added colour to the sunset or a new vista to the heavens.

One of the interesting traits of my mother was her complete lack of materialism. She did not have the remotest interest in possessions and things, and this too was to leave an indelible impression on me.

Children in Europe now seem hurled head first into a frenetic charge of video games, noise, distraction, barraged with adverts and the 'hard sell'. When I was a child, there was no cultivation of the idea of 'more more more'; there was always simply enough. From a very early age, I had an unspoken sense of myself, that it was truly enough. There was in me a private content, and a pleasure in playing with my rabbits in the garden or drawing pictures that no one needed to see because they were for my own delight.

In an ineffable way, a part of me never needed approval or external acceptance. I never felt the impulse to be recognised in anything because I had enough recognition of myself. Perhaps that came gradually, but it was to be a trait of my personality for better or worse .

I was surrounded by animals; every conceivable type of animal. My mother had a rare gift with animals—snails and slugs, worms and bats. We had frogs and tadpoles, rabbits and snakes. We had a spider monkey and lizards. My mother taught biology as well as art, and as a child I remember seeing injured mice and toads and pet ducks following her everywhere. My earliest memory of her was nursing a sparrow with a broken wing. Our garden was always full of frogs, injured animals being nursed, hedgehogs, snakes, rabbits, spiders and beetles. We had stick insects and cats, always lots of cats. Mum told me that birds should never be kept in cages because they were made to be free. She had within her a core of the druidic nature, possessing genuine wonder, marvelling in living things. My mother still has guinea pigs and hamsters, rats and a very large asthmatic black cat that looks like Garfield and waddles slowly. Often in our lives we see birds with broken wings, strangers with nowhere to lay their head, frightened creatures in need of protection, cats in need of a plate of milk.

***

From the very dawn of my life there were many lights that shone, guiding my way. There were people who changed me forever and awoke within me infinite possibilities. The windows of wonder were flung open, constantly, by awesome people who were fully alive. These people would teach me how to celebrate the amazing gift of life.

All of us have those fantasy figures we look up to, and as we get older they sometimes change into other things. Like all children growing up, I had heroes. My heroes were always somewhat atypical though. Most of my friends were into Batman and George Best and, as they grew older, James Bond and The Man from UNCLE. They liked Thunderbirds and soccer players, but I was more interested in what was directly around me. Beside our house there was a retirement home for old missionaries and on occasion I would go and visit them. I was fascinated by the various characters. They were my earliest heroes and made a great impression on me. It was to be my first contact with a new place that filled my imagination, Africa ...

There was one very big old man who looked hundreds of years old, with a big long white beard that went down past his waist. My friends all thought he was Santa's grandfather because he was way too old to be Santa Claus himself. Fr Walsh had ridden into Khartoum with Gordon in 1885. We never understood what that meant, only that Fr Walsh was deaf and blind and had a very friendly chuckle as he sat in the garden like Merlin.

Fr Tom Hughes was only in his 80s, which was young compared to the others. He had been in Uganda, and much to our delight, told stories of the early days in Africa. The thing that I liked most was that his eyes always smiled and there was a warmth in him that was very different to other adults. He didn't seem to know everything and he was much happier than all the other grown-ups. Fr Hughes had spent 20 years in the African jungles and had built schools, and for years he walked through the undergrowth to his missions across the great plains of Africa among lost tribes. He rode a horse from one village to the next until he got a motor bike. I found all this really wonderful and loved the stories and adventures. Fr Hughes also had a mynah bird that could recite the *Pater Noster*, which I just thought was amazing. The old

Mill Hill missionaries in Herbert House were always patient and kind, always welcoming and always, always had the door open. This was something that was quietly leaving an impression on a child's mind, quietly awakening something.

Although I wasn't conscious of it at the time, the happy hours I spent in their company were to have a lasting influence on me, and would shape the decisions I would make many years later in life.

***

In my primary school, Vaughan House, I was taught by a mountain of a woman who never thought like any teachers I was to meet afterwards. Sr Oliver was Austrian, from the Tyrol, and she had a huge influence on me. Like me, she wrote backwards and was left handed. She encouraged me to be myself despite other teachers trying to teach me to write like everyone else. I could write backwards and upside down and always felt happier doing so. To this day my diaries and notes, letters and drafts, things to be typed, are all written backwards.

One morning in art class, I was making a picture of my rabbit Noah, who was a particularly large rabbit, and as I continued off the page, my creation took place largely off the paper across the work bench. The old nun shuffled around clapping her hands with glee at each little masterpiece and then I proudly showed her Noah, my rabbit. She peered a little closer, and then closer still at my expansive bunny rabbit and told me that she thought it was the best bunny she ever had the pleasure of seeing. She turned to the class and said something that has stayed with me always, 'Remember dearies, remember it is never your picture that is too big; sometimes the paper you are given might be too small, but whatever you do, make it as big as you want. Don't stop because of the paper.'

Although I was only seven years old, I remember promising myself that I would never stop at the paper. I was perpetually amazed at the magic of sight and the power to be able to see things. Insatiable curiosity grew within me and never stopped growing. That appetite was to open my heart and awaken possibilities I never dreamt of. I had the most fabulous childhood and felt cherished and wanted. My little victories, pictures and Plasticine, play dough and stories were always greeted with glee by my mum. She always made time to listen to my adventures and the stories from my imagination. I remembered my dreams and would tell them to her, acting them out, and she would be enthralled. I was flooded with love and thought everyone else was too.

It was in 1966 that I went to Bishop's Court. Even though I missed my Austrian teacher, life there was great fun and again I have to say that my childhood in general was absolutely fantastic. My mother had a great sense of humour and believed life was to celebrate. I remember my classmates feeling pressured by parents or hassled by study, but this was something I was never part of.

The school belonged to another age, a different century. It was a delightful, happy and tiny English private school. Such schools for some odd reason were always referred to as public schools yet there was nothing remotely public about them or their pupils. I went there because Mum taught there, but most of the kids were the children of old money, the aristocratic families, some dating back to the Wars of the Roses. It was like those black and white films of schools where there was a graciousness, a dignity.

The school was run by a kindly old gentleman called Mr Burroughs. He retired, selling the school to the Augustinian monks. We were taught about things that mattered: courtesy, respect, honour. There was a strong culture of thinking about others. There were only 120 pupils. I can't imagine a better place to have gone to school. There was no bullying and there was no unkindness that can be typical of boys. People were allowed to be themselves and there was a very English eccentricity to everything. There was fair play and an absence of the pretension or snobbery found in the *nouveau riche*. Nobody boasted about how much land their father had, because there would always be some Indian prince with more. It was never about one-upmanship. We were all too young to be vain and too sheltered to be stressed. I never recall being anxious or tired and I had no concept in me of anger or loudness. I went to Bishop's Court with no clue as to the world that existed outside my realm of happiness, and I was delighted.

I never liked team sports; they never struck me as being very gentle or calm, but ice skating was different and for four years I spent a lot of time on the ice. I also loved to ride horses and would spend hours riding over acres of ground that is now, sadly, an industrial estate. My best friend, Christopher Kenny, was shy and, like me, stayed away from the sports field.

I had a taste for languages and loved reading books about far off places. I read about the jungles of Borneo and the Himalayas and the great cities of the Aztecs. I was, like many children, enthralled by the ancient civilizations long gone and the old kingdoms of the world. It was a world of legends and heroes.

***

I spent a lot of time playing with my growing collection of lizards and snakes, but I was also very interested in adventure. It was then that I started reading CS Lewis, and I would dream of Narnia and Aslan, of the great battles against witches and darkness.

The first book that made me cry was *The Happy Prince*, and it continues to enrich me today. Recently I bought it and sent it to George Bush, and asked him to read it, but he never replied. It is a blueprint of how we should treat each other and think about strangers. Americans are often poor at that. Oscar Wilde wrote such a typically Wildean, fantastic series of stories for children that I loved. There are so many depths to these fables that every time you read them there is a new message. *The Happy Prince and Other Children's Tales* is still, oddly, in the children's section of most book shops. It contains more wisdom and insight than many of the learned tomes in the political science, current affairs, and international sections of these stores. This is a tale about beauty and success, of an amazing life that had never quite been lived, of missed opportunities and tenderness. I remember my eyes filling with tears, reading again in disbelief, again in delight, again in hope. The tale of the happy prince was to remain with me and years later would touch me once again. Each story filled me with something, excited me, and I wanted more and more to know about the selfish giant who finally let the children play in his garden, and the young king who was crowned with love and the beggar girl who was cold and sad. I continued to develop academically. I learnt Latin and French from my father, a linguist. They were my favourite subjects, and I read anything and everything.

I also loved to write stories and poems, and had a few pieces published in the local newspapers.

***

In 1971, our family moved permanently to Ireland, which was a strange transition. We were to continue to travel back and forth between Britain and Ireland during the holidays but the days of the old cattle boats from Holyhead were over.

To this day, my Irish friends are amused by my English accent and my English ones think I have a delightful, soft Irish brogue. Until I was 12 I had travelled between England, Ireland and France. Granny was growing old and the family decided it was time to join her in Dublin. She was a wonderful woman with a big heart. She had survived the Blitz in Liverpool and was bombed twice, but she was unafraid of pain and had a self-possession that I marvelled at. Granny was a milliner but also made the most beautiful dresses. She was always dressed in fantastic colours and was the only one I knew who wore hats. She loved hats and made her own all the time. They were spectacular, dramatic creations that were all very beautiful. Many years later I was to become friends with another creator of breathtaking hats, Philip Treacy.

***

I always loved Ireland and no matter how it changed over the years it has always remained the place I love above all. It is a land of primitive beauty and legend, of myth and music. As I have grown so too has Ireland, in my heart, as a blessing and a light.

The first day at Terenure College was a cultural experience after the rarefied atmosphere of the tiny English school. Bishop's Court belonged to another time, and it was there I was given the most important thing in all education, the inspiration to think for myself. The teachers loved their subjects but also knew there was life outside the classroom. We were taught that what really mattered was not results or academia but how you were as a person. We were encouraged to use our imagination and to create something new, not repeat what was already known. Creativity came from a spark of original instinct and from necessity. Education was about valuing the individual. Bishop's Court had students who, to my faded recollection, were calm and peaceful. Terenure had 700 rather wild and very noisy lads. I was always shy and the drama of moving made me a little quieter. I was always private and self-possessed and sought out others like myself.

***

Tom O'Riordan was from a Limerick background. He was tall, gangly, and ran like the wind. Tom sat beside me on the first day, bowed slightly, and announced himself rapidly in a dialect unknown to me. I stared in perplexity. 'Pardon me?' I said. Again Tomas O'Riordan announced that he was from Michelstown, County Cork but that his father was from Abbeyfeale, County Limerick. After several tries Tom slowed down enough for me to follow him, but his was the heaviest accent I had ever heard. Tom was to become the best friend of my life; my rock, my guardian angel, the one person who would walk with me when things got dark. This shy, self-effacing boy was to become so much to me; the first to unconditionally trust me and believe in me. Tom was the embodiment of modesty and in him I discovered the nature of friendship. In the 35 years that I have known him, we have never had an argument, kept secrets from each other, let each other down, or insulted each other.

Tom is innately incapable of selfishness. He has within him an integrity and goodness that lifts you and protects you. He always had a different journey, but never once faltered in walking at my side on mine. In that time I have never known Tom to put himself first or to be unkind.

His friendship was to define all others and the bond that I formed so many years ago was to lift me when I fell, protect me when I was vulnerable, heal me when I was broken, and sustain me when I had nowhere else to turn.

Tom and I were inseparable from the beginning. I sat by him all through the very happy years in Terenure. Every day was a pleasure and I looked forward to seeing him more and more as the years went by. Because I was born in England, I was exempt from learning Irish, but I was welcome to sit in the Irish class for six years. There I did my homework, drew pictures, distracted Tom and read early history, which I loved. As in everything else at school, Tom was brilliant at Irish. His intellect outshone mine, with never a flicker of vanity or conceit.

I spent a lot of time in Tom's house. His home phone number remains my password on everything to this day.

Tom's mum was the salt of the earth, one of life's givers. From her he was to receive three gifts; selflessness, humility and primal goodness. From his father Tom would receive an unusual intellectual intelligence, a sharp wit and moral integrity lost in modern Ireland. Like most Irish men, Tom was never great at sharing his emotions and found it hard to show physical affection, but what he did have was something else. I learnt the meaning of goodness a thousand times from Tom, and it was during these teenage years that I began learning what being a friend could actually mean.

Terenure College was a wonderful place and I was allowed to be myself. Tom was uninterested in fashion or discos. We were both retiring, both more comfortable away from the crowd. In some respects we were a little odd and our small group of friends would these days be considered reserved and nerdy. Tom was respected because he ran like a bullet and set several running records. He had no technique, style or grace, and like his father's greyhounds he ran with a gangly awkwardness. He frequently accidentally spiked people with his running shoes and on occasion ran barefoot if he forgot his spikes, which was often. Spikes or not, he would still win.

We were part of a group who were interested in Latin and history, maths and the classics. We were by any standard, nerds, but in our comfortable world there was no such thing. There was, as far as I recall, only acceptance. The popular guys like Ed Kelly, Declan Doyle, and Conor O'Kelly were always gentle and respectful. Never was there any unkindness. Tom was considered somewhat rural, but his speed on the track and his rapier-like intellect won him respect. Colm Barry had a rare integrity and dignity, reading encyclopaedias as a hobby, and was, even at school, the highest ranking chess player in Ireland.

English was taught by John McClean, an intelligent man with a sharp intellect and wonderful sense of humour. He taught English simply for the love of it.

For him, English was about self-expression. It was about learning to think in new ways and seeing further than horizons. He read with feeling and taught us to express our feelings, always encouraging us, always showing us over the next mountain. Above all he treated us like young adults: with respect.

I would often write essays about my passions and concerns and his comments were always gentle and supportive, even when I rambled. He was cultivating how we thought and expressed ourselves and was less concerned with the nuances of language. Once I wrote 20 pages about a mystical kingdom that existed in a surreal dimension. The Nobods inhabited this world and lived through dream worlds, passing into the electrical storm worlds far beyond. The kingdom was actually an invisible world that existed in the back of my head. John read every word of this rather odd fantasy, commenting on sequence and style. He took the time to read it thoroughly, and that made a great impression on me; that someone very busy would take time. I felt really thrilled. At the end he wrote one word: 'Wonderful!'

The impact of hearing that you have done something wonderful as a child is transforming. I can think of nothing more important than nurturing children and building their confidence. Words have great power; power to lift, power to crush, power to create and power to bury talents.

I too was an avid reader and had read the Koran when I was young, and thought the 'Upanishads' were a mirror of the 'Song of Solomon'. I gave Tom the writings of Theilard de Chardin when he was 14 and as a result I was considered slightly eccentric as we were leaving school. Perhaps it was the appetite for learning about other worlds, or the extraordinary teachers like Sr Oliver early on, but I was fascinated by everything and wanted to know more. Schools teach things in straight lines, they follow curricula, but I have always been unsure if this was the best approach and my mind did not like moving in straight lines.

While all these friends rose to eminence and success, our lives were intertwined and the bonds formed in childhood are our supports now. One man I admired in school and grew to know over the years was Fr David Weakliam. I also became friends with his nephew of the same name. David was a Carmelite and the head of the school; his nephew was in our class. Fr Weakliam possessed a wisdom and personal integrity I had not encountered before. He was a priest and teacher with a scholastic intellect, a passion for justice and a primordial honesty. Then, as now, his desire to bear witness to gentleness eclipsed all else. His awareness of what mattered utterly touched me in my adolescence at a time when many were becoming sceptical. I remember once David saying in a short, heated exchange with a cynical student, 'It is either that the Christ is God and in Him is all else resting the apex of everything, or that you are right.' I remember those words as if they were carved on my being that day in 1976.

For me that was the ultimate crossroads. Even in my ignorance, I knew that this was the question on which all else would depend. Either that Christ was a historical hoax and deception, or He was the voice and incarnation of love itself and within this incarnation was the undiluted truth of everything. David Weakliam was, and is, a source of that insight and remains a dynamic witness in Ireland of the purity of that message, and a testimony to something beautiful for God. David's nephew was shy, thoughtful, calm, and gentle. He was to become a brilliant doctor and missionary, working for many years in Nepal, changing the way health care was implemented in the mountain kingdom of a strange and difficult people.

There were many things happening in my teenage years. I was learning and absorbing, questioning and awakening. There are many foods for the mind and body, imagination and the soul, and I was tasting them all. The great thing about learning is that you never have to stop.

I had a theory about exams that I still believe. When I occasionally share this theory, panicked parents try to qualify it to children in earshot. My belief is this: the best way to manage the archaic exam system is to not study. The worst thing you can do before any kind of exam is to cram or spend hours reading. The more important the exam, the less you should study. What you should do is quietly and slowly absorb during term, but never write notes. You should only use mental constructs, semiotic diagrams, knowledge trees and acronyms. The rest is like neuro-linguistic programming. The reading you do, if it is done in silence, will remain in your head and be recalled.

More importantly, information is not knowledge. Knowledge is the understanding and internalisation of things. The process of cramming depends on regurgitating information which is not often understood. If you buy into the anxieties of preparing for exams, you join the collective in a shared stress that creates anxiety, worry, changes in sleep patterns, and pressure. People feed off each other's worry and develop mild relief from the shared frenzies. Adrenaline and stress hormones pump through young blood and students have panic attacks. It is much better to go the cinema, swim, play football, dance and enjoy yourself every evening before exams. Another important thing I learnt was to develop in my head webs of relationships that were like miniature molecules and spirals of inter-relationships when remembering complex things. Every night before sleeping I would take time to be quiet, slowing my heart beat, then I would step into the calm of my head and sleep instantly, like turning off a light switch. Tom preferred the study approach, which worked for him, though he was never very relaxed.

***

It was during this period of my life that I began reading the one set of books that influenced me above all others. I read every word that Kahlil Gibran ever wrote when I was 16. I read his books again when I was 17. I was blown away by the power, the force and energy within his simplicity. Gibran was to be the foundation of my beliefs and he challenged every assumption, certitude, arrogance and idea that I had presumed. He was able to speak of all that mattered without pious platitudes, preaching, doctrine or dogma. His words flowed from his heart with tears and laughter. They were not read out of a lectionary or from a theology text, they were alive. Gibran was full of humanity and every time I read his reflections and parables I changed.

From the time I was 14, I meditated. It took a long time to get right. In the first months my mind wandered all the time. I was always getting distracted, hearing sounds outside my head, and returned to thoughts scattered in my head, wandering around uninvited. For months I would practise yoga and breathe calmly. My head visualised but frequently the nothingness was interrupted by the image of a beautiful face, a noise outside, the thought of a sexy body, something I had forgotten. It was not easy. My hormones were kicking in, which did not help emptying the mind. Tennis and swimming were of little help but in time I channelled the new tidal waves of energy into becoming.

I spent a growing amount of time in Cistercian monasteries in Ireland, developing a deep bond with the Cistercian Trappist monk Albert Shanahan. There is a great secret that dwells within the contemplative life. It is a source of interior unity and grace, but that path is not understood in this generation and the ways of inward stillness are not celebrated in this winter.

The places of silence are now only guarded by those who belong to another time, but in time the contemplative life will find new meaning because it is only through our unity with the universe and stillness with our hearts that we find purpose.

Over a 20 year friendship until his death, Albert and I shared our voyage, our contradictions and struggles. I was developing a deep desire for inward stillness, a delight in contemplation and an appetite for silence. Albert possessed something I never had; humility. I had all the certitude that accompanies youth. I had opinions and ideas about everything. The people I admired had focus, insight, intelligence and energy. Albert was always different. There was no ego happening; he had nothing to prove. He taught me that anyone who wants to can hear the inner voice. It is within us all. Outwardly, he was a portly, rather bumbling, goofy sort of guy in bad health, but within him was another world.

The inside of Albert was a universe of blessedness; a tranquility and understanding that I recognised even through the tinted glasses of my adolescent certitude. Albert never once tired of my interminable ramblings on obscure, meaningless theologising. I asked him once if he was concerned about the empty monasteries, the decline of the monastic orders and the aging communities. He told me that there were many ways to celebrate the unknown, and many paths to wonder. He said that light could find its way amid the darkness and that a single candle could set fire to the universe. It took me many years to understand what this meant.

I often went to Bolton Abbey and spent days talking, chanting (very badly) and taking up all his free time, but he gave it gladly, never telling me he was in a hurry; never impatient, always listening as if my words mattered. I learned in time that it was not my words he listened to, but me. He could hear me even when I never knew myself. It was here I first read *The Art of War*, *I Ching* and the *Tao*. I was introduced to the many traditions that had tasted union with the absolute. The ecstasy of Spanish mystics, the fire of the North African mystics, the sexual energies of the Mogul mystics and the abandon of the Rig Veda. I read *The Fire of Love*, *The Mending of Life* by Richard Rolle and the Indian epic, *Mahabharata*. These texts deeply moved me, but it was a short anonymous work called *The Cloud of Unknowing* that blew me away.

Every word of this 14th century manuscript was a new awakening. It spoke of a world made beautiful by our little kindnesses, the language of the other, not of me. It was about our expectations crippling us and hiding our beauty. It was about extraordinary things that lay within us, freed by letting go of our fears. It spoke of the language of kindness that brought a joy that could heal everything. We could redefine everything, become hope, become the gateway, become the journey. We could become the change we wanted to see in the world. We could do this not through knowing but unknowing, through drawing closer to what matters beyond words and thoughts. *The Cloud of Unknowing*, like Kahlil Gibran's poetry, radically altered my self-realisation and awakened within me a very new awareness.

Over many years Albert cultivated within me a disposition of quietude and of stillness. Once I told him I would love to be a Trappist like him, and he chuckled and smiled at me. He told me that my path was elsewhere and that the monastery of my stillness should be in my heart, in my head, and in my body, but above all in my spirit. It was on one of these many retreats visiting Fr Albert that I met Molshie.

Molshie Walsh was a short, passionate Passionist nun from Kildare and our energies embraced each other long before we did. Molshie was unconditional acceptance personified, and saw through my childish verbosity straight into who I was, and delighted in it. I began a friendship in the late 1970s with Molshie's extended family who were untouched by the crap of civilisation. In those days in Ireland there were still many communities whose lives were free of the materialism already changing Dublin. The thing that was most magical in Ireland was its people. There was time to talk, time to listen, time to be present, and there was a genuine pleasure in sharing the little we had.

Advertising and media played no role in their lives, a farming people who were the salt of the earth. It was here I had my first lessons in people being Christian first, Catholic second. There was a simple faith with basic values like charity, humility, kindness, giving, forgiving, caring, serving. It was unconscious complete acceptance at a tribal level where all cherished all. The cultural leap from South Dublin to the Walsh clan was far greater than the gap between the Western world and the Nomads of southern Sudan who ran around starkers and had huge spears and lived in mud huts. Nothing prepared me for the welcome, generosity and warmth of Molshie's family. I would often spend weekends just drinking tea and going from home to home, always embraced, hugged and made to feel like one of the family. I remember thinking that if I ever had my own home it would be like theirs; a shambles—full of stray cats, dogs, ducks, chickens, children of every description, no airs and graces, but a kitchen teeming with life, a magnet to everyone who wanted to feel at home.

There was an old lady who came every day for her dinner, not a relative but sucked into the family, with never a hint that it was from kindness. It was nothing of the sort, it was simply Ish being Ish and Paddy being Paddy. Paddy was a huge mountain of a man. While not exactly metrosexual and never having seen a mirror, Paddy was, above all, selfless.

And so it was; my unlikely heroes began to form ranks within my subconscious. The snob in me had been silenced by graciousness, and the Toms, Alberts, Molshies and Walshes had awoken something in me, something fed by silence, enriched by reflection and touched by angels.

CHAPTER TWO

'I like your Christ, I do not like your Christians. Your Christians are so unlike your Christ.'
- *Ghandhi*

Many influences mould young minds. I grew up in an unrestricted environment where we were allowed to be ourselves. It was a time free of the political correctness of today. I was always affectionate and open but I fear we are creating a generation of children who are nervous of affection, inhibited and on guard. The influences that moved in me were a synergy of traditions; art, music, ideas and cultures. The secret of wisdom is to know our own inner child and celebrate the dance. Growing up, we develop our minds and bodies, souls and senses. The peculiar thing is that we sometimes think we have arrived somewhere. It's only when we become awake to the magic of life that we see it's only just beginning.

1976 was an important time. Mao died, and I felt relieved for China. I felt excited as the Viking probe landed on Mars. Everything was new and inventions were happening all the time. We had the first digital watches that no one could actually read because you pressed a little button and somewhere there was a faint red digital read out that couldn't be seen in the sun, but we thought they were fantastic. We felt very modern compared to our parents with their 30 year old watches. In 1977 Elvis Presley died, Apple computers went on sale and chaos hit New York as looters went crazy after Manhattan had a blackout. We were amazed by *Star Wars* and by everything else we were discovering. And as with the new awakenings all around, I had my first crush, somewhat behind everyone else's. Her name was Therese. The nearest I got to her was playing tennis, which I did exceptionally badly. The only one worse than me at tennis was Tom, whose approach was to whack the ball as violently as possible in any given direction, which occasionally led to bodily injury, generally mine. We were really crap at tennis and Therese soon discovered Brian McCarthy, who was very trendy, good looking, and played tennis better than Therese. I would point out to her that the wooden tennis rackets belonged to Tom and were very old while Brian had a silver graphite racket that looked a lot bigger than ours.

I often wondered if ours were actually early squash rackets but Tom assured me they were once used for tennis. We resigned ourselves to the fact that we would not be future tennis stars and went back to cycling in the Dublin Mountains. We went swimming and hiking. I lamented the loss of Therese, though my energy turned to keeping up with Tom, who cycled up hills with legs like pistons and the determination of an early Celtic zealot.

There were many influences that were awakening new possibilities and dynamic energies that stirred in my heart. Somehow, deep down, my future life was forming within me, but I didn't yet know what it was or how to allow it to take shape.

In 1977 I met a man who was living my dream, although I was too young and self-preoccupied to understand it. Jean Vanier was a Canadian, a gentle and kind man who had seen the needs of the vulnerable in Canada and did something about it. He created a community that would care for the emotionally and mentally challenged. This was not easy and he overcame the odds to achieve it. Jean Vanier was in Ireland and I heard him speak. He had founded the International L'Arche Community, which works living with the poor and rejected people of society, and his talk had a big influence on my own way of thinking, really highlighting to me the difference between the haves and have nots.

In the late 1970s in Ireland there were no jobs and most of my friends began slowly leaving for studies, opportunities and relationships abroad. Tom had started medical college and I joined *Les Pères Blancs D'Afrique*, the White Fathers of Africa. I was 18, and very much drawn to what they stood for. They came from a French tradition and I spoke French, and they worked with the poorest of the poor. They had a humility I never possessed, which drew me closer. I love French and absorbed the energy, passion and vitality of the dynamic group who lived to try and make a difference in Africa. Eugene Lewis was the Provincial of the Order and reminded me of Captain Kirk in *Star Trek*. He had a huge heart, an innate common sense, a deep grasp of people, and knew what really mattered. It was 1977 and already cracks were appearing in the Catholic church, with dissent, gender issues, attitudes to other faiths, and other issues all being debated. The old power base of the Catholic hierarchy was replaced by smug fat cats in BMWs who were about as spiritual as a used car salesman, and it was starting to show. As Ghandhi mused, 'I like your Christ, I do not like your Christians. Your Christians are so unlike your Christ.'

***

Jesuits were above all free thinkers, often far outside the constraints of convention. They have challenged orthodox ideas for centuries. The missionaries I was with were very different. Some still had recurring malaria and others were broken by the diseases of the jungle. Some had gone very strange. One old man mumbled to himself in a forgotten African language, while another, caught in some massacre, was waiting for attackers to come through the roof at night.

I had been reading philosophy since I was 11, but the more I read, the more I realised I didn't know. So when I finished school, I decided to study philosophy in the Jesuit Institute in Milltown in Dublin. The world was sweet. There was time to think, to read and to reflect. I was surrounded by people who shared the same hope and ideas and searched for the same thing. There was an openness; radical and political ideas were challenged and explored. It was new and there were movements across the world questioning the status quo.

For me, philosophy was what made the world work. Most people, I felt, had stopped thinking. This is even more so today. Philosophy means becoming what you can be, what you have the potential to be, by challenging yourself, and not simply adopting the vegetative state of accepting what is in front of you.

I have always been worried about certainty because in its worst forms it is approaching evil. The certainty of George Bush, or the Taliban, for instance, is dangerous. We need to keep asking ourselves questions because nothing is ever certain. Even at the age of 17, this was clear to me, and it naturally led to my interest in asking the big philosophical questions, the big 'why?'

Philosophy for me wasn't about reading theories, it was about reading the thoughts of visionaries throughout history, who stood up and asked the world why, throwing out insights to better humanity. This could come in the form of ancient cultures, mystical texts, artists, anybody.

There are a lot of misunderstandings about the subject. We need to teach people to think, and philosophy is about beginning this process, about being awake, surprised, aroused and amazed. Philosophy is life. Your life, my life, all life. It is everything. It is how you live, not Heidegger or Kant, but something exciting that opens us up to the world and all its ideas. Poetry, art, music—they all come from it. It is simply how we are, the harmony made up of many differences that gives the world a dynamism that triggers questions, that in turn make us ask more questions again.

My small class began questioning our own responsibilities and the individual exterior and how we related to it. Our comfort zones were broken and many of us were asking the same questions. Who were we and why did we need these man made structures to be loving or caring? How loving and caring were we in systems that were out of touch with peoples' lives? We spoke about the sick and the lost, the lonely and depressed, we just never met any.

The class was made up of several religious orders: Carmelites, discalced reformed Carmelites, Passionists, Jesuits, Dominicans, Oblates, Servites, Sacred Heart missionaries. Even then the distinctions between the once great monastic orders of medieval

Europe had vanished. The reasons for the foundation of the old contemplative and mendicant orders were only remembered by scholastics and ecclesiastical historians.

While some of us, myself included, were fascinated by the evolution of early medieval traditions, others were more radical. There was already movement across South America calling the Church to be more open, more in touch with humanity. The public face of the Catholic Church had become stuck in act-centred moral issues. Its media and pastoral agenda was preoccupied with condoms, divorce, sexual morality. Liberation theology challenged the complacency of the hierarchy and the winds of change were bringing new ideas to a generation of young clergy. The Polish Pope entrenched orthodoxy and there was a gradual rise of intransigence. Right wing groups like the Legionnaires of Christ and Opus Dei found new favour in Rome and gradually liberal movements and left wing bishops were eclipsed by those more in line with Rome. Of 24 people I knew well in Milltown, 20 would leave their orders to express their calling in ways less constrained.

Life among the White Fathers was never boring, always exciting. One member was a young African priest, who in a way different to ours had a devotion and a closeness to the invisible. He would kneel straight in the chapel transfixed in prayer, in the dark, and would always serve us, always be attentive to us. I remember once being late climbing over the back wall on a cold winter's eve, sneaking into my room. There was a knock on the door. The young priest bowed gently and passed me a huge mug of hot drinking chocolate, thinking I might be cold.

On another occasion I was sitting alone in the library. My hand had been very badly burnt a few weeks before and I was afraid of the operation to come. Covered in bandages it had been bleeding and I was in a lot of pain. I was self-conscious because of my loss, as I was completely left handed in thought and character. I rested the swollen, bandaged lump on my lap and was just sitting there trying to deal with the throbbing mass of pulsating pain shooting up my arm. I remember that moment thinking, 'Shit, shit, shit, damn, stop, stop . . .' and little else. The nerves were destroyed but somewhere there were bolts of undiluted pain firing violently through me. There was water in my eyes as I opened them and the young priest whose name I now forget was kneeling there in the semi darkness. He lifted my swollen, heavily bandaged mess in both his hands very, very softly. The bandage had seeped a little and I was embarrassed at the blood and yellow stains. He kissed the bandaged mess at the end of my arm. He said in French, 'I pray to take away this pain and carry it for you, I pray only to feel this moment with you and I thank God that I hold your hand here now,' and he bowed his head. When he raised it, his eyes were full of tears.

My hand developed a thick purple scar that became a large lump like cold purple wax that was stiff like a frozen slab of meat. The scar gradually grew into the artificial tendons, and this caused growing concern. The consultants advised that my skin was hypersensitive and was prone to keloid growths. A keloid is a thick raised overgrowth of dense scar tissue. This large angry looking scar covered the back of my hand and looked like purple rubber. It had no sensation. The doctors were worried at the prospect of the tropics for such reactive skin. My friend Michael MacGreil suggested the Jesuits might be a more fruitful path, and soon after getting my degree in Philosophy I entered Manresa and the Jesuit Novitiate. I was by nature drawn to solitude and inner stillness and the radical politics of many Jesuits challenged convention, disturbed complacency and worried Rome.

I had never believed in an absolute truth or one way to being real. There are many paths to living a life of gentleness and few of them need labels or words. It always seemed to me that the only thing that mattered was how we reached out to each other. I just did not quite know where to begin.

Pedro Arupe, the head of the Jesuits, spoke of radical witness and service and of the poor. Morris West's epic, *The Shoes of the Fisherman*, told of a Pope who would come from the oppression of Eastern Europe, a man who had been in the Gulag, tortured and held in solitary confinement. In this novel, the humble, very human man who ascended the throne of Peter understood the people who were struggling as best they could to find some meaning, some sense to it all. Ireland was already changing and by the time John Paul II landed to a monumental welcome the Church was already crumbling from within. Neither Rome nor the Irish clergy would be prepared for what was coming. The charismatic Pope was a holy man, a gentle man, but so rooted in medieval Christianity that he had no comprehension of ordinary currents of thought. Surrounded by sycophants and pious clerics he was shielded from the mounting storms that fell on an institution bereft of light.

The Church was so disconnected from what people thought that initial responses to breaking scandals remained smug, condescending and hypocritical. Many of those who provided assurances turned out to have been living many lives. Within a decade the mask slipped and Ireland was revolted and disgusted. In time revulsion became anger, and anger cynicism, a condition that suffocated innocence and blinded many to all things spiritual. Religion is not what men have made it, nor is it the edifices we fill with altars or images. It has always been elsewhere. The failure of church men in every civilisation is that they often cease believing themselves and one day the people see that there is no light in the eyes of their priests and no fire within their hearts.

The sadness of man made institutions is thus; they are born from the fire and inspiration of free spirits ablaze with Love. In time these dreamers find followers, and the followers make rules. The rules become laws and the laws are held as truth, and in time the laughter of joy is replaced by the coldness of certitude.

Francis, the Umbrian mystic, was such a child of light. Francis was young, beautiful, and full of life, born to merchants, loved by many. He followed a dream which brought him to cherish the lost and unwanted. Francis gathered a few friends and together they lived a simple life believing that Christ came into the world as a poor man to serve and give, heal and be gentle. Francis drew criticism from the wealthy monasteries but in time those who followed him were in their thousands. By the time he returned from the Holy Land his order had become wealthy and the custodians of his dream had become indistinguishable from the orders Francis had sought to be apart from. Francis went into the Umbrian hills and in his stillness found deeper union with the invisible.

He received the stigmata; his mysticism had been drawn into a different dimension of ecstasy. Francis, who had given his bed to lepers and cherished the broken and unwanted, now rests in the splendour of a magnificent tomb in Assisi, his witness to the poverty of Christ celebrated on gilded altars. As Zitkala-Sa said, 'A wee child toddling in a wonder world, I prefer to their dogma. My excursions into the natural gardens where the voice of the Great Spirit is heard in the twittering of birds, the rippling of mighty waters, and the sweet breathing of flowers: if this is Paganism, then at present, at least, I am a Pagan.'

In the 1970s an American Jesuit, John Powell, had written a series of books which were about living our lives to the full. The titles themselves were inspirational: *The Secret of Staying in Love, Why Am I Afraid to Show You Who I Am?, A Reason to Live, A Reason to Die*, and a book written about his spiritual journey, *He Touched Me.* These, together with the writings of Ghandhi and Einstein, were opening within me new ideas. The Torah and a lot of Eastern Vedic writing all seemed to spring from the same well. The mystical traditions at the heart of the human race spoke with a single voice. Whatever about religious traditions and institutions, our relationship with the Sacred seemed to be free of the clutter that clogged up churches. The idea of the middle path in Buddhism and of cherishing creation in the 'Upanishads' seemed very familiar with the ways of enlightenment in Jewish and Islamic meditations. The wisdom of North American spirituality reflected Guru Nanak who founded the Sikh religion, drawing the spirituality of Islam and Hinduism together. The Benedictines Dechanet and Bede Griffiths had shared the close bonds between monastic contemplation and Raja Yoga. The Cistercian Trappist monk Thomas Merton campaigned against the Vietnam War in the 1960s. He was a poet and theologian who wrote beautifully on the mystical paths of the Eastern and Western traditions, their freedom and unity. The wisdom of other traditions was drawn together for a new generation by Anthony De Mello, an Indian Jesuit who wrote many books about awareness, becoming, discovering. There were mostly collections of Eastern mystical parables, fables, stories and tales. While the Vatican was unhappy with many of these thinkers, people were listening, asking their own questions and finding their own paths. Many people began to look beyond the confines of the world they grew up in and began exploring other ideas and cosmologies. The day will come, I hope, when humanity will not be divided by religions but will share a common spirit and be part of the love that will make us whole and to the light that will guide us all home.

Life is big, very, very big. When we are caught up in these microcosms we can miss the majesty and vastness of the universe. There is a Blackfoot saying, 'What is life? It is the flash of a firefly in the night. It is the breath of a buffalo in the wintertime. It is the little shadow which runs across the grass and loses itself in the sunset.'

It explodes into life creating all around it freely from its mighty forces and meridians of being in countless forms. All around us are birth, rebirth, becoming, writhing, teeming, dynamic synergies from atoms to the heaving of the cosmos, miracles exploding across the abyss filling the darkness with light. When we think further than ourselves, we start to see with new eyes, new vision. It was in a moment of reason such as this, awoken by my own stillness, that the tiny seed of an idea sprang to life within me. The idea was simply letting go of my own fears and doubts and trusting more in this energy within.

***

I was befriended by an American Jesuit, Corbett
Walsh, while in Manresa. Corbett was from Boston
and had that long slow lilt that lets each word softly
touch the next in a melody. Corbett was in his late 40s
and was on sabbatical. For many years Corbett and
I were to write to each other and share our journey.
He was the first person I ever heard talk of Jesus as
if He was a man. Albert Shanahan was in union with
the invisible, a mystic united to the sacred, touched
by the divine, illuminated by something not of this
world. Albert walked with angels and saw into the
miracle. Corbett was more like me, a man wrestling
with the paradox, struggling with a Church out of
touch, challenging himself and torn by the bloodiness
of humanity. When Corbett spoke of the Christ, he
spoke with such incredible tenderness and wonder
that I was always transfixed.

On one level he worried about the petty things in
life. He was bothered by syntax, disturbed by details,
irritated by people and annoyed by hypocrisy. But
whenever Corbett spoke of this man, he raised in me
a desire so great that it burns within me now brighter
than ever before; searing, intoxicating, overwhelming.
Corbett taught me more than my years in philosophy
ever could. He opened my eyes to a raw truth; that
Christ had nothing to do with institutions or churches,
and everything to do with me. The frail, vulnerable,
very little me. One evening we were talking about life
and death and how we would like our epitaph to be
written. The younger we were, the more pretentious
we were, and then it came to Corbett, and his eyes
were full of tears, and he nodded his head gently and

he whispered the epitaph he would want. His voice was tender and barely audible . . . that 'he was kind'. If in a life a man can be remembered for this alone, then all of life's chaos, all the cruelty, all the pain and all the turmoil would be worth it. For in kindness is incarnated Love. In it are the graces of acceptance and mercy, and the graces of compassion and selflessness. None of us receives as much kindness as we should and certainly we could all do with more each day of our lives.

To me then and now, this spoke so deeply to my inner flame that it grew into a raging furnace. I can see no better way to spend a life than in pursuit of this, the most momentous and epic of all ambitions—to be kind. Corbett gave me Nikos Kazanzakas' *The Last Temptation*, which was one of the most transforming books I have ever read. In our long conversations about it, I began to realise that humanity was the unveiling of gentleness, and greatness came from tenderness. This epic novel was about ultimate becoming; becoming love, becoming one within each other. I became increasingly excited at the possibilities of being able to live everything within my imagining, and by the awareness that there were no limits apart from those people teach us to believe.

Ireland was a strange place and most of my friends had left, flying to the far corners of the world seeking their fortune. There were few jobs in the late 1970s. There was a despondency which was in ways the lull before the storm. It was a tempest that would be a catalyst for change as we wrenched ourselves from the perplexed grip of a Church that had lost its people.

I was increasingly interested in Eastern mysticism. The Western traditions too held secrets so powerful that I began to question the direction of my life. The extraordinary examples of love and courage were all around us. I kept reading so many things that inspired me but I was changing in my own life. One night I re-read a medieval text called *The Imitation* by *Thomas à Kempis*. They were gentle and simple words, disarming in their simplicity, and they touched me as no philosophical or metaphysical writings had. Like the Lebanese poet Gibran, these words written in the late 1300s had a power that transcended everything. A Kempis wrote a rare understanding of love as incredible internal power, a power that would change the world. Here is my own translation of one tract:

> Love is a great thing, powerful above all other things, which alone makes every burden light, and equals every inequality. It bears the burden and makes it no burden.
> Love wills to be raised up, and not to be held down by any meanness.
> Love wills to be free driven by gentleness and being united, lest its inward power of vision be hindered.
> Nothing is sweeter than love, nothing stronger or more powerful.
> Nothing will heal you more or free you more completely.
> He who loves is in wonder and ecstasy.
> He gives all things for all things never measuring what he gives because he rests in the inner light.
> As the same fire assumes different shapes when it consumes objects differing in shape, so does the one Self take the shape of every creature in whom he is present.
> Love has no measure and will overcome all the darkness within and around.

It strives after more than it is able to do and does not see the impossible. It is unstoppable and succeeds never being overwhelmed despite the brokenness of the world.

Love is watchful, though fatigued it is not weary, though hurt it is not destroyed, though alarmed it is not terrified, but like the living flame and the burning torch, it shines bright and heals.

If a man loves, the fire of all love is within him and he is never alone, never angry. He belongs in the invisible and is held by it.

May I learn this love, may I learn to taste with the innermost mouth of my heart how sweet it is to love, to be dissolved, and to swim in love.

Let me be filled by empathy going beyond myself,

Let me sing the song of love, let me follow joy, let my soul exhaust itself amazed in the light of love's wonder.

Love is swift, sincere, in awe, exciting, gentle, strong, patient, faithful, prudent, long-suffering, perfect, and never seeking its own; for whosesoever seeks his own, there he falls from love. Love is forgiving, humble, and tender; not weak, not fickle, nor intent on vain things;

never fades, free, raw, quiet, and wise.

I knew I had to open my eyes and challenge my own direction. There is a cynicism that has an artery into our psyche in Ireland. At its best it throws us G.B. Shaw and Brendan Behan, awakens in us new thrusts and energy. At its worst we can be begrudgers, and we can mask our cruelty with the thin veils of a humour that diminishes and demeans. There lies within our national disposition a tendency to reduce each other and pull down, a negativity that has in our past been a nihilism which has not served us well. It was healthy in this winter of thought to leave Manresa, to follow the example of so many and spread my wings.

CHAPTER THREE

'The most beautiful thing we can experience is the mysterious.
It is the source of all true art and all science. He to whom this
emotion is a stranger, who can no longer pause to wonder and
stand rapt in awe, is as good as dead: his eyes are closed.'
– *Albert Einstein*

It had struck me as somewhat odd that people could
sell hours from their lives for money. The concept
of work as a social idea never seemed reasonable
to me. It meant that people would surrender their
waking day for money. This money would go towards
building a nest and preparing for the future, towards a
few weeks' holiday and the preparation of children to
earn money too so that they could sit in places selling
their time as well. To my mind there just seemed so
many other things I should explore and uncover. It
was time to step back from education; it can interfere
with learning.

There are many intelligences, many dynamic
paths that illuminate our way. My heart drew me to
open my mind and be less analytical. Einstein said
that two things were infinite, the universe and human
stupidity, and that he wasn't so sure about the universe.
His religion consisted of a humble admiration of the
illimitable superior spirit who reveals himself in the
slight details we are able to perceive with our frail
and feeble minds. My own needed to be challenged,
awoken.

***

I was fortunate enough to have some family wealth at my disposal and was able to travel around Europe with friends in what I would now call 'the beautiful life with the beautiful people.' I always loved skiing and spent a lot of time with friends in the Alps. I had known many young Italians and French friends from Annecy and Mont Blanc to Aosta and Torino. I knew the French and Italian Alps well, and gave skiing lessons to pay for my upkeep. I had places to stay in Grenoble and Cuneo.

I enjoyed teaching girls to ski because they were more relaxed than boys, and had less of an ego to bruise when they slipped. The first girl I kissed was Italian, from Milan, and I had met her on one such trip. She had dark brown eyes that sparkled and lips that were soft. There was an innocence to her embrace and a purity in her touch. Francesca looked like a catwalk model and she laughed from her heart at my jokes and said things that made me feel good. We spoke in French and she laughed in Italian; she filled my thoughts and invaded my sleep. My skiing friends were mostly French and all were excellent on the slopes. Some of my friends worked long hours on holiday; I sunbathed. and trained most of the time.

I had practised yoga since I was 12 and it developed my body as well as my mind. By the time I was 17 I was ripped with very defined abdominal muscles. On one occasion in Marseilles I was asked if I was interested in being photographed. I declined, but after a second offer I began doing body art modelling. It was nothing like face or catwalk modelling, it was mostly black and white artistic shots of shadows and light. I thought it somewhat silly to photograph a back or a shoulder or a torso, but the funniest bit was being paid for it.

Every summer I did some fitness photo shoots, mostly body photography, arty stuff, and in a few hours I made more than my friends earned in a week in their summer jobs. The work allowed me to travel around at my leisure, spend time with my friends, and enjoy life. I always thought it was a far better prospect to be handed money for standing still rather than working. It was funny because people I got to know through modelling began to believe it was their beauty that was wanted by the photographer, not realising they were only the raw material. I had already grasped that appeal and magnetism were about energy and self-possession, not how you pouted your lips or flexed your body. It had not dawned on them that looks were fleeting. Vanity is always comical, especially when taken seriously.

I fell in love with Paris at an early age and there was an innocence in discovering the simple delights of long, lazy afternoons in the parks, or exploring the galleries and backstreet cafes. We had parties and met artists and writers, photographers and musicians. French and Italian kids were very different to my Irish friends. The pace of life was more to do with being present to each other and drinking was a calm, unhurried sipping of wine.

I sculpted and I skied, explored France with friends and moved from one great city to the next. We discovered galleries and parks, museums and tiny cafes. We meandered in Tuscan villages and cycled country lanes. My friends Francesca and Raphael were in ecstasy with every exhibition and their insatiable appetite for art electrified us all with a contagious enthusiasm that had no boundaries.

They were calm and intelligent, sensual and awake. Raphael would drift between long tender embraces with his girlfriend to arguments about where his eyes wandered in supposed infidelity. Such explosions were so deliciously Italian that I relaxed into their moods awaiting the passionate reconciliations. They were to marry and have many children, each wilder and more fiery than their parents. Tasting life became about opening myself to the possibilities beyond the walls I had been building for myself. France and Italy were about deconstructing my own fears and habits, trying to let go of myself for a while. It was natural and the energy of Calabria and Tuscany only awakened in me other passions and tastes unknown and unexplored.

***

There is an old African saying that I only understood after many years living in the bush. *Journeys never happen in straight lines and time is never divided into equal parts.* We white people often think in boxes and divide life into segments; we are taught to think in straight lines, a habit unhelpful to artists, inventors and most humans. Humans are creatures best suited to living in their hearts, but these days too many leave far too many important things up to their heads.

I would visit Tom when he had a break from university. Here I was; I had this amazing life, rich with friends, each of whom illuminated my life—I had everything anyone could want. I sat on Tom's bed in Terenure and told him that if we had all this, if we had such a fantastic, amazing life, we should perhaps share it, because the fantastic life we had was not in itself enough. It would be a great idea to see others have what we had. Life was even more awesome than before and possibilities came from every direction; there was a constant sense of the now and how exhilarating things were. Just when we thought things could not get any better we were stunned by some other discovery or adventure, experience or pleasure.

Siddhartha Gau-ta-ma was a prince who lived in great wealth. He was protected from the sufferings and needs of his people in much the same way as the happy prince in Oscar Wilde's short story. Siddhartha, so the legend goes, one day left his palace and explored the city outside. As he passed through the city, for the first time he saw tears and poverty, he saw cruelty and need. In his journey through the streets where his people lived he discovered not everyone lived in delight. Siddhartha Gau-ta-ma followed a journey of discovery and through it became enlightened. He died in 483 BC and became known as Buddha. The examples of Jean Vanier, the Mill Hill priests, the challenges of Ghandhi and the rise of poverty across India and Africa had presented an exciting opportunity.

We had television and we could not say that we were unaware of the poverty and need in our world. I could not pretend to myself that everything was okay, nor could I say it was someone else's job to reach out to the hurt. I felt very deeply that it was up to each one of us to do something to make a difference. A few pounds in someone else's collection box would not do it. Paying someone else to touch the frightened was not enough, I needed to try and do something myself, to leap out of my comfort zone and find out where and how I could do something that could change someone's fears and pain. It seemed a very obvious idea.

I looked at my life and realised that I had so much, so I began to think that it would be a great idea if other people got to have as much, or to share what I had. It was a child-like aspiration, yet it is at the heart of all humanity.

I suggested that I might to go and live with the poorest people on earth. I had not figured out how, why or where, and was not remotely confident that I myself made any sense. I was half-hoping Tom would convince me that this was a rather unsafe, unwise and scary idea but instead he just was his typical self. 'I think you should. That's a great idea. How can I help? What can I do?'

There was always an unconditional, undiluted belief and acceptance in me from Tom. The rest of the world might have thought I was silly or wasting my time, but not Tom—he always believed in me. I think you can always do the impossible as long as there is someone, somewhere, somehow, who despite everything, believes in you.

Within me was the tiny, frail, delicate and fragile seed of an idea. It was very weak and could so easily have been destroyed. In those days the slightest damage would have killed my little dream, unspoken even within myself. Here this tiny flickering flame of an idea was guarded, not just by me, but by Tom, who protected and encouraged me, though he knew not the why or the wherefore. He only knew that he believed in me. I only knew that this seed would tear asunder my life, security, safety. It would separate me and hurl me somewhere else. I was afraid, I was unsure, I doubted myself but not the dream. I trembled, but only from my fears and the ghosts around me. I wept, not for the poor but for myself at what I was doing. I was uncertain and unclear. Within me were the images of the BBC, Brian Barron's reports from places far away, Malcolm Muggeridge's documentary on Calcutta.

There were the photographs of wasted, frightened children, mothers crushed by grief, desolation and lost futures. I remembered Ghandhi's words, 'An ounce of practice is worth more than tons of preaching. Be the change that you want to see in the world.'

On the other hand there was my life and everything I knew. The beautiful cities, secure suburban life and beautiful friends who were gracious, fun and intoxicating in every way. I was drawn, I know not why, to trying to change the way we were looking at extreme poverty. It seemed very distorted. The images that reached the media have not changed in 40 years. The skeletons of the Biafran War are identical to those in Samburu today and the withered children of Somalia in 1980 are the same icons taken by digital cameras now. I was never a zealot, and never wanted anyone else to live my dream with me, but at the same time I did not want anyone to take my dream away from me. I never had an idea of giving up my lifestyle, I just thought it would be worthwhile to live two lives, perhaps many lives.

***

We are distracted by an ever increasing deluge of information. Now, more than ever, we are flooded with facts and data posing as news. This is often in the form of the frailty of celebrities, the latest accidents, tragedies and political tensions. Media thrives like vultures on misery. Others, like the Lords of Poverty, as I call those who make a business of it, depend on it and even benefit from it. The reaction to human misery seems to be divided into several forms. There is the genuine heartfelt desire of ordinary people to try and reach those they see suffering, the aid industry or multinational businesses spending billions in development, and most dangerous of all, the political games of rich countries using aid to further their own agendas. In the 1970s the German Chancellor Willie Brandt produced a challenging blueprint for change. Like all attempts to change the way we thought about the poor world, it would be debated, discussed and reviewed. After all that's said and done there is a lot more said than done and when the rhetoric in front of the cameras was over the Brandt report became forgotten, remembered only by academics and librarians.

With all the influences I had had, and all the thoughts that had developed over time in me, I became more and more convinced of what I wanted to do. I knew for sure that I would never be able to work towards a conventional career, or work for other people, to fit neatly into society as a nine to five man who came home from the office to his semi-detached home, wife, and two and a half kids. I just wanted to live my own dream, on my own terms. That dream involved connecting to my innermost spiritual beliefs which, though I was still young, were strong.

I wanted to live my life in a way that showed that I loved joy, that I celebrated life and connected with everybody else on the planet, sharing the good fortune and whatever wealth I had, be it actual or spiritual. I wanted to love this man, to live as he had instructed; this Galilean carpenter who had the only idea of any major philosophy or religion that made sense—to give everything we have to each other and to treat each other as we would like to be treated ourselves. This to me was not following religious teachings, it was following common sense, and my own instincts.

I kept thinking about the story where, after the Resurrection, Peter came to Jesus to talk, and Peter said that he loved him. Jesus asked if he really loved him, to which Peter replied that he did. Jesus asked the same question again, and Peter gave the same answer. Peter then asked, 'How can I show you that I really love you?' Jesus replied, 'If you really love me, you will go and feed my sheep.' That was it for me. It all made sense. I always dreamed of feeding the sheep.

But I didn't really fit the spiritual model, or the medical or charity one. I wanted to live my dream but on my own terms. At one stage I thought it meant becoming a priest, but I realised that was just feeding my ego, making myself out to be a holy man. Then I thought that perhaps it meant living my own life as I had so far enjoyed it, in a hedonistic, fun-filled way; leading a life filled with sex, art, good friends, good food, and a certain amount of luxury in a privileged sub-set. Every one of my friends in France and Italy was like a sex fantasy, and I could very easily have settled into that lifestyle of luxury and sensual living.

But whereas I knew this was open to me, it just didn't feel like the right option. To be honest, all I wanted to do was to ski, have sex, and enjoy life, and that has never changed, but I don't do it because I knew then and I know now that there are more important things to do in life.

If I was going to be honest with myself, the only thing I knew I wanted to do was what I ended up doing, and that was helping the poorest people on the planet. I wanted to leave a footprint on Earth, and I wanted to do what I saw I needed to do. I also wanted other people to look and realise that we should all be doing this, but as a starting point, I had to begin with myself.

I have never lost my connection with that world of models and skiing, beautiful people and beautiful surroundings, and every now and then I visit old friends who still live that rich lifestyle, but now have their own homes and families. I will never have a house, a car, or personal wealth, but I can still ski, drink, party, and most importantly, live my life, which costs nothing but is the most precious thing.

I realised I didn't have to give up everything I knew; that I could go and help the poor and still lead a separate life. I could have all the things I enjoy, but I could still feed the sheep.

***

I started to become very interested in finding ways to deal with poverty and global health and wrote an article about it for the *Irish Medical Times*. I still knew relatively little about it, and went to see the editor who was ready to help me. He suggested I go and see the grand old man of tropical medicine. He told me of a man who had been involved with the leper clinics in West Africa in the 1940s. Joe Barnes was practising in Nigeria and the Congo before the days of charities and NGOs, was at the start of Concern, the Tom Dooley Fund and the Refugee Trust. Joe Barnes was a legend and his name was known across Asia, the Middle East and Africa. Joe's Doctorate was in leprosy, even before the days when they could properly treat it. Joe had seen more lepers than every doctor in France in the leprosy clinics combined. He had performed surgery on the pygmies in the jungle, been shot at, bombed and attacked. Joe was the first medical doctor working with the medical missionaries and was among the first in the killing fields of Cambodia. He saw the conflicts between organisations in camps but also the heroism of individuals and the dignity of the few.

So it was that I came to see this legend who had done so much, leading only by example. Joe looked like an old druid, a Gandalf or Merlin without the beard. He was tall and his face bore the lines of laughter. I was given an Irish welcome; a firm handshake, and brought by a great stone hearth where Joe listened to what I had to say. I don't actually remember what I said, though I must have talked too long for Joe started to doze. I was not quite sure if I had bored him into slumber or if he was just drifting off. The thought briefly crossed my mind: *what if he passed away while I was boring him?* Finally Joe opened his eyes and smiled. His eyes always sparkled and he told me that it was a great idea and he would be delighted to help. The idea was simple enough. Tom, Joe and I gathered a few more friends. Kevin Niall and Des McCabe had both been in our class in Terenure, and together we began our little community for the relief of starvation and suffering.

We would create an African vision for development through the dreams and ideas of Africa without imposing our own plans. It seemed to me that there were a lot of wonderful Western organisations with very Western agendas that fulfilled vital roles, yet there were not enough driven from traditional beliefs owned by Africans. The plan was to go to Africa and see if this idea was workable. If it was, then we would try to find ways to support it.

We needed guidance on the next step and I went to London to visit some of the leaders in international health. I started with a friend whom I had written for and already knew. Ian was the editor of *The Lancet*, and he introduced me to Gordon Smith, the head of the London School of Hygiene and Tropical Medicine.

Gordon, like Joe, belonged to a generation of pioneers who reached the top, dragging everyone else behind them, in the days before cut throat competitiveness. Theirs were the days of gentle graces, when people had time for each other.

I would often visit Gordon for tea and he would introduce me to the nutritionists and physicians who had shaped much of the thinking in tropical health since the 1940s. These were men like John Waterlow and Hugh Jolly. There were the Professor Joliffe's and Woodruffs whose names filled library shelves, and then I met David. David Morley remains one of the most loved paediatricians in the world. His work in maternal child health changed generations of doctors across the globe. David was the first professor of tropical child health in the UK and he pioneered the role of mothers at the centre of health care. He greeted me with the passion and enthusiasm of a fellow pilgrim. David had a huge department, with dozens of projects across the world, but he had a tiny desk in a small box room. He had given his office to his students. If he was given a new bag or chair he would pass it on. He was never one for trappings or prestige, and his humility was exceeded only by his kindness.

We had now gathered the necessary expertise to guide our steps. David had spent decades in Africa as had Joe Barnes, and now it was time to venture into my dream. I had been blessed by knowing many people who had spent their lives in Africa but nothing prepared me for what was to come. David Morley was the inspiration for generations of health workers and was loved. Everyone he met he helped and guided. He understood that health was about well being. David always saw the big picture and believed in people. He trusted them. He had an inventor's imagination and imagination has always been more important than knowledge. Einstein said that 'a person starts to live when he starts living outside himself'. Guided by this small band of wise men, I officially set up ICROSS, the International Community for the Relief Of Starvation and Suffering, and after months of planning, we were ready to begin.

CHAPTER FOUR

'You may not be able to do great things, but do little things with great love.'
– *Mother Teresa*

Joe, Tom and I had developed contacts with old missionaries in the Karamoja Desert of Uganda and in the Turkana desert of Kenya bordering Ethiopia and Sudan. Joe had known many of the Irish missionaries, being the leading specialist in tropical medicine for many years. I knew a wide network of Irish and French missionaries made up from friends in *Les Pères Blancs*, as well as Italian contacts in Uganda and Somalia, many of whom I had met during my first visits to Florence and Turin.

I went to the Karamoja. It was the poorest place on Earth and was in the grip of a savage famine that was ripping life from children and burying tomorrows. It was the height of the famine. I had been sheltered from human suffering all my life, only reading about it and seeing it on TV. The experience of coming from the comfort of a jumbo jet and hours later seeing human beings subsisting with absolutely nothing requires the creation of new words. We use language in reference to the known, we describe and narrate to each other on the basis of common meaning. But what do we do when the experience falls so far from our comprehension that it is outside our map of what is?

The first thing that strikes you in the desert is the relentless sapping heat that is like a hammer in your head, draining you, with no air conditioning, no cold water, no place to step away. The second thing is the all-absorbing and tangible dryness that hits your eyes, your lips, your tongue. The desert has its own smell, a sort of dry, dusty, oppressive smell, and its own harsh energy.

I have been in six famines but always remember the first vividly. My first days were full of this self-preoccupation with physical conditions; the dust, the wind. The heat had its own sound as it microwaved the earth in this desolate melting pot of nothingness. The Italian nuns had been there many years and continued their work long before the cameras arrived and long after the media went home. I remember the sweat seeping from me, first hot, then cold, then hot again. I was soaked from morning to night. It was only after the first few days that I began to get a hold of my own body and its distress in this new world. I had been so busy with the climate shock to my system that I had not yet started opening my eyes and learning.

One evening I went with one of the old nuns to a little hut; no more than a few twigs curved together. We squatted in the half light and the old nun knelt beside a small grey blanket. As my eyes adjusted, I realised that it was not a blanket on the earth but a young woman and at her side a tiny child. The woman's breath was laboured and shallow and the old nun whispered in Karamojong long into the night.

She tended the child and wrapped it. As the moon rose in the sky I could clearly see the shivering, dry, grey body lying in the dirt, the old nurse at her side. Before we left the young mother gave her last breath and Maria brought the infant to the clinic.

For weeks I explored the Karamoja, moving from mission to mission in old land rovers belonging to missionaries, writing cheques where I could from money raised through friends and family. There was a lot of money, and I handed it out at every opportunity until there was none left and I had gone heavily into debt, but there was never going to be enough to go around, never enough to stop this desperate situation, and in the end I felt impotent, useless, unworthy to be here in the midst of desolation. I felt a raw sadness outside of myself and a dawning of anger began in my heart.

There were so many great people doing so many wonderful and important things. Above all I noticed the kindness of mothers for the children of strangers, the gentleness of children towards each other and the dignity of the old who had seen these things before. The thought awoke in me that if I was struggling here, what were these children doing? I had a bed and a mosquito net and was drinking water all the time. What was it like for a small child who had utterly nothing on this earth, in this place? I followed the famine to Turkana, landing in Kenya.

I was collected by Paul Cunningham, a Holy Ghost Priest with over 40 years of experience in Africa. Paul was one of those people who always left everyone he met changed—richer, happier. Paul immediately held both my hands, beamed brightly and gave me a big hug. When you are alone, arriving for the first time in a strange place, there is nothing more wonderful than being befriended so completely. Like a lot of the old missionaries, Paul knew both the culture and language. His network extended throughout East Africa. He was to create ICROSS in East Africa with me and was to be my mentor until his death 14 years later.

If the Karamoja had been my initiation, Turkana was to be my education. The Turkana are an ancient people, old even by Africa's standards, and they have lived in the unforgiving northern deserts for centuries, their ways understood only by themselves.

The first thing I did was to start learning the Turkana language from a blind boy called Arawachan. My teacher in everything else was a medical doctor from Dublin who had spent 35 years in Africa. But Robbie was no ordinary doctor; Robbie had entered monastic life with David Weakliam, giving himself to the Carmelite order. He had nearly died from TB as a young man, and had always suffered ill health. He had recovered, became a renowned physician, represented Ireland at Wimbledon, spent decades in Zimbabwe and was now living among the oldest of the ancient warrior tribes.

I remember one occasion in Dublin with a smile. Robbie looked older than Dr Joe, but was still to be seen in Fitzwilliam Lawn Tennis Club. A hot young seed was looking for a game of tennis. He was in his 20s, Robbie nearly 60. Robbie, always self-effacing, was volunteered. The young buck felt eager for any kind of game and was kind enough to take the bent over, bald old man on to the court, not knowing who or what he was. Robbie, hunched and small, always posed a deceptive opponent, and many had made the mistake of measuring him an easy game. Straight sets later the young seed had been wiped from the court with Robbie's praise for a great game, and a week later he had returned to the Sub-Sahara, while the young player went on to great success.

Robbie welcomed me as a brother and never once showed a moment of assumption that he had anything worthy of sharing. He had everything I didn't, he was everything I wasn't. I was blessed with every step I took, with the giants who had moulded the way in which tropical medicine was understood. Above all I was graced with people who taught me simplicity. Their wisdom had generated in me a humility that was not innate. I saw in the Paul Cunninghams and Robbie McCabes something I had never grasped; humility.

'Paulo' was venerated, made Elder by the leaders of the Kikuyu. His name itself was a passport and he was loved by the poor and the powerful. He said Mass in the most dangerous slums and at the same time visited the mighty.

Robbie shared everything he had and did so unconsciously. His ultimate delight was to listen to opera. This was always a surreal experience in the midst of the desert, with Robbie deeply sensitive, modest to the point of self-oblivion, and yet gracious and resolute. To use the word 'kindness' in relation to Robbie would be a gross distortion of language. Everything that Robbie did and does is about other people and how he can give to them. From the second I met him I was made to feel that my contribution was critical, that I mattered and that everything I personally did was essential. It was this important doctor who had spent his life simply in the service of the least and the weakest who taught me a primal truth. *Whatever you do, live by it forever.* Robbie belongs to an order of mystics: John of the Cross, Teresa of Avila, and simplest of all Therese of Lisieux, all burning with the same elemental connection to what matters above all else: Love. The missionaries running clinics and hospitals in the most remote places had been among the people working with them for decades. Their experience and wisdom, humility and connection, was amazing. I was to see that dedication in some 26 African countries I was to visit and work in over the following decades. Across Africa and Asia there are thousands of unsung heroes toiling away unnoticed and unacknowledged. I was touched by the welcome in every mission. These were not tired, burnt out or disillusioned people. They were passionate, on fire, inspirational.

***

The problems faced were immense, and they kept growing, expanding, throwing out scenes and situations that would stop any person in their tracks. I was walking on the shores of Lake Turkana one morning when I came across the half-eaten body of a child lying on the pebble beach. To see this once can raise feelings of horror and dread at how cruel and uncaring the world can be, but the tragedy was that this would never be a one-off scene. The same week we were walking to a village when we found the remains of a child who had starved to death and had died clinging to a small bush. Her eyes were still open, staring into the distance. The image was devastating.

That week I was introduced to a young Somali called Bare Ali Sheikh Mohamed Abdi, and he was to become a friend who would work at my side for 30 years. Bare never believed in work and thought white people were sad because they thought too much. He was the first person I knew who could do everything in slow motion.

There was gunfire at night because the Merle tribe were at war with the Turkana, and this made the situation even harder to bear. There are tribes that have fought for centuries for reasons often forgotten. Such conflicts were now reduced to cattle rustling. Bitterness runs deep and vengeance to those who have not tasted it is baffling. People are capable of great cruelty and meaningless destruction.

The village was behind barricades and fences of thorn trees. I remember being angry as I saw a tired woman whipping a young child over and over, while others stood around and watched. I ran over and snatched the stick from her and shouted at her in a language she would never understand. The child was bleeding and for the first time I experienced meaningless cruelty. It tasted sour and bitter and smelt foul. I told Bare to take the child to the clinic. It was not even this woman's child, but an orphan who had been trying to steal a small, stale piece of bread. That evening I told Robbie about the horrible woman and the apathetic people and the bleeding child. I was annoyed at his own response at not sharing my rage. Robbie had treated the child and found her a home. I had just become angry. I was learning every day.

The desert was, however, so vast and still that it eclipsed even the violence of the few and welcomed me with a calmness. Much later Robbie shared in passing that he had always found ways of placing his sorrow and emotions into healing and useful things, because anger would never help that child or give her bread or clothe her, but perhaps a quiet resolve might.

While I was being culture-shocked in Africa, Joe and Tom were quietly gathering support in Ireland. A group of friends in New York were trying their best to help as well. A Holocaust survivor had read a description of the famine in *The Lancet* and had written to me. This small group of people set up ICROSS East End (of Long Island) and were to become partners for over a decade.

The article was a few stories of the poverty and conditions, but it had drawn interest. The secret of all victory lies in the organisation of the non-obvious and I set out to find the shortest possible path to it. Lord David Owen had referred to the article in Parliament and I made the journey from Uganda to Westminster to see him. I had been in the bush for a long time and had worn the same shirt most of that time. My sandals were more worn than most and I had not cut my hair. Looking back, David Owen was quite right to tell me to go home and get a hair cut, as I was a disgrace. I was, however, given tea by Edward Heath who was a gracious and kind man who talked a lot about Beethoven and Wagner as well as taking an interest in our work. We needed people to take an interest, but we also needed them to help in every way possible.

***

In the first few years I tried to learn as much as I could about health programmes in Africa and Asia. There were many opportunities to travel and learn from those who were doing real work and had great experience. The Flying Doctors, AMREF, became good friends. Sir Michael Wood, the founder of AMREF, and his family, provided great encouragement and support. We were to work side by side with the Flying Doctors for many years.

Many of the students of David Morley and the School of Hygiene and Tropical Medicine were now in key positions in health care across the world. One invited me to India to see how primary health care worked in the slums of Bombay and Calcutta.

In those days Calcutta was always humid, full of a putrid, vile stench and suffocating still heat that fills your breath like an asthma attack without Ventolin. It is crowded, pulsating and pressing with life, but in the heaving mass of people there is a poverty that cannot be wiped clean. The tiny lanes between the slums are full of excrement and the streams are putrid, with garbage everywhere. The air is oppressive. It was there I first met Mother Teresa, already revered and canonised by those that matter. Like many visiting the slums I went to the headquarters of the Missionaries of Charity and had not searched long in an open ward before the tiny busy presence of Mother Teresa appeared and welcomed me. I was to meet her three times.

I had gotten lost and was on a street crowded with merchants, stalls, cows and rickshaws. The humidity was like being in a steam bath, the sweat so thick it was coming up my nose. I stepped over the puddles towards the main street. There was a line of beggars, old and young, hideous and scary. There were children with no hands, others burnt, and others with growths. There were lepers with eaten faces and heads looking like masks. It was a surreal place and I was distracted by the tingling of sweat dripping down my back and the pulsating of my head in the stench. I was making my way to the end of the sorry row of the destitute when a girl called out amid the noise. I no longer remember what she said as I was too preoccupied keeping myself out of the mud. This young woman in the dirt signalled at me, and to this day I still do not know what made me go over to her. She asked me to take what was clearly her child.

Words were few and mingled with a harsh guttural tongue but the message was apparent. She was asking me to transport this child to the clinic. She did not know if I had access to any clinic and I do not know why I stopped. I had walked by so many beggars with my head bowed. I thought of helping but this seemed to me to be a very bad idea. But it was a decision made in one of those instants so easily dissected afterwards. Whatever the reasons, I ended up some minutes later in a rickshaw with a strange woman and jumping the queue in a crowded clinic run by German nuns. I remember feeling my heart pounding inside my body, knowing I had left my comfort zone and sensing in myself that I really should be somewhere else. Anywhere but here. I attached myself to a large European nurse who had an air of authority and hurriedly explained what had happened. I had left the somewhat spaced mother in the rickshaw and had carried the moving bundle to this person who was clearly in control. She was a kind woman, capable and gentle. She humoured me and took the child. I was so relieved and my fear was replaced by a different anxiety. Something was seriously wrong here. I was ushered to the corner of the examination room and shown some soap. I used it all and most of a bottle of antiseptic. I felt a mixture of revulsion and annoyance at myself; part of me was disgusted by the heat and smell, another part of me grossed out, but I was unequipped for what happened next.

The nurse was giving instructions, calmly and softly, to the assistants around her in Bengali. I noticed that the assistant had started to wrap the infant in plastic, and the body was moving. It was moving strangely, though I did not understand why. The young nun was very kind to me though I was tired and uneasy, and I wanted to go. I did ask her what was wrong with the child and I saw the mother being taken into a side room by one of the other local nuns. Everything smelt very bad.

She brought me by the hand to where the infant was flinching on the large examination table. She opened the child's tiny mouth and said something gently to me but I don't remember what she said. The child's mouth was full of worms. The little girl had been dead a long time. And was being eaten by intestinal worms.

I do not remember leaving the clinic or saying goodbye. I only recall the sense of being out of my depth, in a place I should never have been, afraid and uncertain. I felt scared but I don't know why. I felt angry with that mother and with the people around me and with everyone else. Above all I was angry with myself, but I had no idea why. I felt way out of my depth, wondering how I had drifted so far from home. I had nothing to offer, nothing to give, and felt overwhelmed. I had a strong sense that anything to do with all these things was best left to nurses and doctors, professionals and the religious groups that were so good at helping the poor.

Some part of me resolved to return to Europe, possibly continue raising money when I could to help. My mind drew me towards what was safe and familiar. Suddenly I missed Paris a lot and Dublin even more. I wanted to be with my friends, talking about the latest film and the new art exhibitions. I did not want to see any more squalor or human misery, it was just too much to witness. If I could reach for the TV remote right then I would have changed the channel, but I didn't and I couldn't.

When we are faced with essential things we either embrace them and are transformed through them, or we ignore them. Whether it is the grief of great loss, the pain of being unwanted, or being the victim of violence, we choose our response and determine forever how it will shape us. When we see tragedy or cruelty, injustice or evil, it is we ourselves who will determine the 'what next?' I was reminded of

Einstein's reflection, 'A human being is a part of a whole, called by us—universe, a part limited in time and space. He experiences himself, his thoughts and feelings as something separated from the rest ... a kind of optical delusion of his consciousness. This delusion is a kind of prison for us, restricting us to our personal desires and to affection for a few persons nearest to us. Our task must be to free ourselves from this prison by widening our circle of compassion to embrace all living creatures and the whole of nature in its beauty.'

Within me, there were many paths to choose from. Right about then the cafes of Paris and the exhibitions in Milan looked pretty good. Soon it would be the skiing season. Modelling was out as I had not been training but I had been invited to Rome and to a course in Sydney. I had perhaps seen more than I intended and got more than I bargained for. ICROSS had become a tiny little group with four health projects in Africa, and had given small grants to a dozen others in Asia and South America. Because of our size we had no overheads and our Dublin office was Dr Joe's home.

We had done what we set out to do. Our efforts had been our contribution to the crazy madness that was hurting people all over the world. It was enough. I wanted to do my sculpting, and dance again. I wanted to teach beautiful girls to ski and flirt with them and laugh with my friends and swim in the sea. I wanted to get ripped again and look sharp, I wanted ... I wanted.

CHAPTER FIVE

'The big things are what you do with your heart.'
- *Lemoite Lemako*

I was torn, torn by all my wants and by what might just be an improbable but necessary quest. Francis Thompson captured it in the epic, 'Hound of Heaven':

> I fled Him, down the nights and down the days;
> I fled Him, down the arches of the years;
> I fled Him, down the labyrinthine ways
> Of my own mind; and in the mist of tears
> I hid from Him, and under running laughter.
> Up vistaed hopes I sped;
> And shot, precipitated,
> Adown Titanic glooms of chasmed fears . . .
> . . . Heaven and I wept together,
> These things and I; in sound *I* speak—
> *Their* sound is but their stir, they speak by silences . . .

Reason called me one way, my heart another. There were many parts to my life—there was a private inner self, the child that was me. This was woven of my ego and humour, imaginings and appetites. It was my creative self. This me was the playful, wild and instinctive spirit that was curious and passionate.

There was also me as us, the close group who were my delight. Some were in France, others in Ireland and England, as well as scattered across the Earth. They were my me, and Tom, Joe, Paul, Francesca and the others brought me incredible pleasure and delight. It was all a gift, all magic.

In my heart of hearts I had no idea what I should do, but I knew I should do something. There were many currents of thought at the time. There was no anxiety but there was an anticipation. Giving part of me was clearly not enough, as simply giving money was not enough either. I was reminded of the story where Jesus told a follower who had asked what more he could do to follow him, and Jesus replied that he should give away all he had to the poor. My heart knew that to believe in something, and not to live it, is dishonest. My mind was made up.

***

I returned to Kenya and with the help of Fr Paul and my friends there we registered ICROSS in Tanzania and in Kenya. With the Director of Medical Services guiding us, we identified some of the poorest areas with the highest mortality rates and most extreme poverty. We were going to set up disease prevention, child survival and water projects. It was very exciting and with the wisdom of the old men who guided me, my enthusiasm was always tempered with their good sense. The Holy Ghost Fathers had always encouraged the learning of the local tribal languages and it was a path that was to become vital to all we did and do.

I went to live among the Samburu Nomads in the Northern Deserts. I always believed that the importation of Western ideas did not work. There is a colonialism at the heart of many well intentioned efforts to help others. They are children of a lesser God in many ways and the model of Africa I felt had become poisoned. The imagery we grew up with was of the helpless Blacks being saved by the Whites, of young, tearful nurses in t-shirts bearing the logo of a charity, holding crying, starved black infants. The message this sends about the charity does raise funds to do important work, but the message it sends about Africa and African mothers becomes embedded in our perceptions and we find ourselves with a caricaturised perception of a pathetic, helpless continent. In part this has been the creation of the very charities working there. The child cries because it has been lifted from the arms of its mother into the hands of someone who cannot speak its language. The mother is not important for the picture and so remains off camera. Unless the mindset that has dominated charity in Africa changes, the model that governs response will remain unchanged. This charity model has been altered and professionalised since Biafra, yet in the present famine that has spread across a million miles of East and Central Africa, the images are the same and the appeals for pity and support compete to a public that has grown tired of tragedy, fatigued by the barrage of marketing and paid street fundraisers. There is a growing scepticism about an industry that has become a good career option. This was true in 1980 and even more apparent nearly 30 years later.

I met a man who lived life full on. Jame Leadisimo was a bull of a man, a Samburu warrior with no fear, a great heart, full of passion. Leadisimo was magnificent and worked with us in our clinics. Like the wind, sometimes he was there, then he would vanish, and months later return with his infectious humour and gentleness. On one occasion a man tried to stab me and steal our ambulance, but he left minus three of his fingers thanks to Leadisimo.

Another time there was a raid and rustlers attacked a tiny clinic looking for drugs they could sell. Leadisimo, with two other Samburu, charged a gang of a dozen, putting them to flight in a gladiatorial display Hollywood would not dare try, returning covered in blood, self-possessed, purring like lions after the slaughter. He had barely broken a sweat. Leadisimo did not have the delay system most of us possess, the 'what if?'. The raiders had escaped, but at a price, and they would not be back.

***

I met incredibly influential people wherever I went, and when I least expected it. One night during torrential tropical rains we went to a homestead. There was a young boy there who was very ill, burning with fever. He was more drenched than Leadisimo and I who had waded through the storm. Lemoite nearly died of malaria. He never really belonged to this world, having always been more spirit than human. Lemoite became my first adopted son, given by his father as he had so many. Lemoite Lemako was the soul of the Samburu, a very old spirit, comfortable for a while in a body. Lemoite has never been concerned by the things most people think about and his inner peace shone from every pore of his being. The Samburu, like the Maasai, are nomads, and their way of life, though vanishing slowly, formed me over many years. It was like living in another century or on another planet.

He was half Rendille, half Samburu, and he remains the human incarnation of calm. Lemoite means 'he who is everlasting', and in him there dwells an ancient soul, connected by light into the very heart of goodness. He always radiated a peace that silenced others, stilled angry dogs, made loud people listen. An old man once told me that Samburu meant 'the people of the butterfly', but that Lemoite was part of the first spirit, and last spirit, and was of the other world. People who have never met Lemoite think we exaggerate or romanticise him, until they meet him. Many years ago I brought him to Ireland and we appeared on a TV show with Pat Kenny, talking about the life we led in the Northern Deserts. Lemoite was simply himself, a primordial light on us, a presence at one with the now, an energy complete and intact with itself, so wholly possessed of himself that he is harmony in human form. He once told me that everything we do should be as if it was the very last act we ever do.

Over the years we have had many Japanese volunteers through a scheme run by the Government of Japan. One was a woman who had worked with us for two years. Before she left Africa, she told me that she was a Buddhist and had all her life practised Zen, but that Lemoite, in himself, was Zen.

For many years we kept camels and goats, donkeys and cattle which we gave to families as they needed them. Every few years we would restock herds and strengthen the bloodlines where we could. One day, I asked Lemoite why he was always so peaceful. He did not understand the question and after I explained it carefully in Samburu he looked at me with his magical smile and thought for a long time. After a few hours still walking with the camels we breed, he offered a thought. Lemoite spoke. Here's a direct translation: 'If you belong here and know you're here, then you're here, but maybe if you think you should be somewhere else you won't be here, you'll be two places, here where you don't want to be and there where you'll never be.' He went on: 'People think too much and their brains get too full and there's not enough space left to stop thinking and be what you're meant to be, thinking only for little things. The big things are what you do with your heart.' Then he was silent again for a long time, totally at peace with the Samburu Great Rift, the camels and the sunset.

Lemoite still lives among us in as much as such a spirit can be here. He is in Seketet, north of Maralal where his people have dwelt for centuries. He is in the famine but not of it, fighting the drought but not perturbed by its devastation. He wipes away tears, but does not become them, and tastes poverty, transcending it with a dignity that can only raise us from our knees and lift us to the stars.

***

Our life in the bush was simple in a way that it was for us before the Romans came. It was in many ways primeval. There were no toilets, no toilet rolls, no seats, electricity, roads, and there was no post, no clean clothes, no sheets, no slippers, nothing we think of as familiar or cosy. There were no reference points. At least none we could relate to. There were fleas and there were lice sometimes. We did have those. There were bed bugs but no beds, and flies in swarms. Flies were so dense that in every homestead then and now the children's faces were covered in them, thousands of them in their ears, on their eyes, in their mouths, thick and fighting with each other for places on little noses and sores.

The huts were made from cow dung and were small and dark, heavy with smoke, without windows. And yet they were always teeming with life, laughter, giggles. The one thing that hits visitors between the eyes all the time is the joy, the relentless bottomless unending celebration of everything all the time. In a land so full of suffering and poverty, it truly is a gift to find such joy in the surrounding world. I remember talking to an old nun in Somalia in the midst of the civil war. She was running a clinic in a vast remote wilderness and had been there for 30 years. I asked her what were the most enduring impressions she had from being there.

She thought, and then thought some more, as gnarled, stiff fingers wiped her brow. 'The people, the children, the laughter, just so much delight in life, delight in everything . . . yes, the people.'

We grow up with expectations and often these become our desires. Even when they are met we take so much for granted. When we no longer understand what enough is, we slowly lose the plot. We collect more, then still more. When our homes are crowded with these things, we buy newer things, upgrading, updating, getting the latest, fastest, biggest, most powerful. When we do not understand the concept of enough we become trapped and this is a type of poverty because it is hard to escape. We become conditioned to think that even when we have three pairs of shoes we actually do really need more.

***

Life in the bush is always full of surprises. In my first year I was bitten by a scorpion, chased by an ostrich, had a camp demolished by elephants and came very close to a messy end swimming in Lake Turkana, unaware of the crocodiles silently watching, only metres away.

I remember one occasion when I was sleeping in the bush. It was hot and humid, and the dawn had not yet come, but shafts of light were threatening to dart across the sky in thin bolts. I felt a weight on my body, a moving mass that smelt of red earth. My consciousness flooded with adrenaline. I caught a breath and woke up with my mouth filled with living, moving things. I was covered in ants, millions of very big black ants. There were so many that I could hear them, which was not difficult as they were in my ears and up my nose. They were in my hair, trapped in my beard, down my neck, up my arm. They did not start biting until I moved and then they all bit at once, everywhere. Sarune thought it was very funny and calmly tried to help, Lemoite sat up smiling, unbothered by the few ants traversing his legs, and I went into a sort of jumping motion which only further entrenched the now angry legions that were clinging onto every millimetre of me. Having flung off what clothes I had, Sarune brushed off hundreds of ants that fought back. By the time we finished I had been bitten everywhere and an hour later the scratches and itches had swollen. I decided I didn't like ants but ants were positively pleasant compared to other adventures with leeches and lice.

We lived in small cow dung huts in Maasailand and Samburu. We would have an open fire on the ground in the middle of the hut and usually five or six of us sitting around it. There was no electricity and no radio, no running water—only containers brought by donkey.

Sarune belonged to the spiritual lineage of his people. His father, Ole Lengeny, was very old and very connected to the invisible. Everybody took this in a very matter of fact way and there was no incantation, trappings or ceremony to it. It just was. Sarune often had dreams. Sometimes he would share them, but rarely. As he was cooking the tea early one morning he told me he saw an old Indian woman in one of his dreams and she was walking through flowers in a big park that had trees and she was covered in blood. I thought nothing of it as his dreams were often cryptic. It was 28 October 1984. A few days later, Indira Gandi, the Prime Minister of India, was assassinated by her own bodyguards while walking in her garden. Over the years there were many such examples. We know so little and our knowledge is so limited, it is easy to understand why the wise are humble.

In the beginning we would do mobile clinics on foot, zig-zagging across the plains and Rift Valley from village to village, simply because we didn't have the money to pay for cars. In Samburu we went through the undergrowth. Lejiren, Leadisimo, Lemoite and other warriors would come with us, each with hunting spears, elegant, beautifully crafted throwing spears, much longer than the heavy war spears of the Maasai. Sometimes in Marsabit and Turkana we could see on the plains raiding parties crossing the floor of the Rift Valley in the distance. In those days the warrior tribes still carried spears but by the early 90s they would all be heavily armed. It was a surreal, unhurried time. We could have been living a thousand years ago. However, all things are in dynamic transition and the old ways were already changing. The tribal languages were known only in the Interior, and within a generation they would all but vanish, with only the old knowing them. The beautiful poetic and mystical depths of the Nilotic tone dialects would be replaced by a pidgin

Swahili, peppered with English and Bantu-abbreviated words. The dream world would be transformed as vast tracts of land would be fenced off and urbanisation would spread to every town and trading centre.

Once, in Uganda, after our car had broken down on the road, we crossed a small river on foot, heading to a village. It was dusk and the village was not far, so we waded up to our waists in the still water. Our guide was from the village and assured us there were no crocodiles. The bridge was ten miles south and the water was clear and still. Four of us crossed easily from bank to bank, which was less than ten feet across. By the time we were near the village I felt a sensation on my back and thighs. In was only in the half light of descending dark that I felt it, then another: wet slugs on my back. They were small and felt sticky. The others were in traditional cloth that they had taken off crossing the river, but I was in t-shirt and trousers. The torch was flat, and it was getting dark, so I stripped and Bare, the Somali from Turkana, felt for each leech. There were a dozen. We finally made the village and I sat by the welcoming fire. An old woman reached over to my neck and removed another slimy, sticky leech that was sucking my blood. They were hard to feel, as they secrete an anaesthetic to numb you with, leaving them free to gorge themselves on your blood while you sit there none the wiser.

The next day we got a lift from the local school teacher who had a donkey cart and we crossed the river by the bridge heading to a main road so we could hitch to the nearest town. Under the bridge on the bank of the river, were three large sleeping crocodiles.

I remember rowing a tiny rowing boat on Lake Naivasha; Paul was busy fishing and we found our-selves surrounded by hippos. Now it might be worthy to note something about hippos; the hide alone can weigh half a ton, and they are the third largest living land mammal, after elephants and white rhinos. They are 13 feet long, five feet tall, and weigh up to three and a half tons. They can move very fast in water and can turn over boats. Hippos are very aggressive and territorial, and can go psycho at the drop of a hat. They have developed some ritualised postures but the huge open-mouthed 'yawn' that reveals formidable teeth is one of the most aggressive. With the long, razor sharp incisors and tusk like canines, the hippo is well armed and dangerous.

Hippos move easily in water, either swimming by kicking their hind legs, or walking on the bottom. They look stupid but they are deceptively cunning. With small ears, eyes and nostrils set at the top of the head, they look placid. These senses are so keen that even submerged in water, the hippo is alert to its surroundings. By closing its ears and nostrils, the adult can stay under water for as long as six minutes. It should be noted that more people are killed by hippos or buffalo than by lions.

A baby had come up under the boat and the females charged us, thinking we were a threat to the young. We both broke into a cold sweat as a dozen tons of hippo launched themselves 20 feet from the rocking boat. This boat was a tiny wooden two-seater and Paul, ever calm, suggested we retreat and not hit the calves too hard on the escape route. Our escape was hampered by another young hippo entering the fray, by which time a large female took a bite at the oar. This was six feet from us and while the fishing rod fell overboard along with Paul's hat, I made a good attempt at breaking the world rowing record in a toy boat. The hippos were still in pursuit as we widened the precarious gap, when I noticed Paul setting up another fishing line. I was ready to collapse but Paul was all ready to try again, apparently unfreaked by our near demise moments earlier. I did learn three things that morning: how to row very fast, how to catch fish with a hook and a piece of string (and it did taste great!) and eventually, how to take anything that happens in my stride, to recognise that the world can change in an instant and can be filled with fear and joy all at once.

We were often joined on our safaris by Tommy O'Sullivan. Paul, the Maasai and I would often go for long trips into the bush. In the 1940s Paul was a hunter but now he was armed only with a childlike curiosity, binoculars and an extraordinary knowledge of wildlife. What he did not know the Maasai did and their connection with their land was always amazing to watch. I never cease to be in awe of their wisdom. As the modern ways have transformed new generations, the old ways are rapidly being forgotten and many Maasai children these days can only talk Swahili or English. This is a real shame.

Tommy was a brilliant man, funny and wise, with a rapier-like intellect. He would always have a fresh way of looking at a problem and a different approach to ideas, memory and meaning. He lived with childlike abandon and was enthralled with people, always ready to give you his time, his space, his energy. Tommy died on his motor bike late one night after a night out with friends. He was in his seventies, always ready for the next adventure, always up for a mystery trip.

***

Every few weeks a few of the Maasai warriors and I would drive into Nairobi to St Mary's, the headquarters of the Holy Ghosts. I was strangely delighted when Fr Paddy Leonard said I should one day be buried with them in the little graveyard. Paddy was the head of the order and was also on the board of ICROSS. He was a really great human being who never let systems get in the way of people. Paddy, like Paul, had an open house. We would sit on the veranda and plan our next safari. Paul shared the old building with Fr Pearse Moloney, who was a stoic and holy man, conservative and self-disciplined. He was always very kind and caring. Once Miriape, a six feet two inch warrior, brought Paul the skin of a leopard, but the cleaners stole the claws and teeth. Another time he brought Paul an 18 foot python skin. He was unlimited by convention and belonged to the people of Maa, not to Kenya.

One evening Fr Pearse proceeded in his bathrobe to the bathroom as was his schedule, and as he walked the corridor he was passed by Miriape, stark naked, resplendent in his nature. Fr Pearse never made the bathroom and retired to his room, never raising the matter again. The Maasai loved Paul who was made elder of the Kikuyu with colobus monkey robes long since stolen. Paul once told me that you should always get up and leave Africa the day you are no longer amazed, and my God, he was always in awe of life, and with his arms open wide he embraced everyone who came his way. Paul had established many schools in Kenya. Nervous young kids would meet the headmaster and be greeted with this amazing smile and a welcome fit for the Christ child.

The only things that interested Paul were whether the kid was happy, what he enjoyed most, and what he liked to play. He understood human nature, but above all he understood what mattered and lived it.

During big school events he would often be seen leaving the compound on the back of a motor bike driven by Major George Whidey. George was the lover of Lady Michaela Denis Lindsay. Michaela was fabulous but completely barking mad. To film historians, she and her late husband Armand were pioneers in wildlife filming even before television came into vogue in the 1950s. She lived in a world more fantastical than any science fiction. I have been in Elton John's home talking about AIDS in Africa, but even his self-portraits on the wall had nothing on hers. Michaela was like an elderly Bette Davis on speed. I was once asked by Cardinal Otunga to go to one of her seances as she claimed one of her spirit guides was a 15th century French Catholic monk and I spoke both Latin and French. The experience was so surreally off the wall that I had not the heart to hurt her, though Michaela believed with all her heart that she was conversing with Napoleon, Martin Luther and a female Pope who died in childbirth.

***

As I travelled across the globe I met many great characters and eccentrics. Africa and India are full of them, individuals with their own unique world view. In recent times these are being replaced by photocopied people with the same perceptions, ideas and thought processes.

Americanism in true *Dilbert* fashion is mass producing mediocrity so that people actually think they are interesting, thinking what everybody else thinks, echoing what everyone else has read in the paper. The media offers insights as challenging as a soundbite and political correctness trains originality out of us. Terms like 'anti-establishment' and 'unconventional' become derogatory in a society free of innovation. 'Controversial', once considered a prerequisite to creativity, is now a condemnation.

The culture of mediocrity gives rise to celebrity, with people famous for being pretty without actually having done anything other than look beautiful. In such a society there are no Socrates's or Einsteins, and no place for heroes—only images. It is on this 'popularism' already choked in its own boredom and disposability that media thrives. New religion is the illusion of success by virtue of adulation and the adoration of form that does not exist without Photoshop.

***

ICROSS was working in tribal areas that had never received any health services. With the help of the Irish Government we began building dispensaries and clinics in remote areas inaccessible by road. The first of many important clinics we built was in Shombole on the Tanzanian border in an area of extreme poverty and endemic tropical infections. In 1985 the Ministry of Health worked with us in Shombole and we immunised over 80% of all the children in an area where no one had been immunised before. Many Tanzanian Maasai began coming to Shombole for treatment and in 1986 we built the Enkare Naibor clinic in Tanzania. There were huge problems facing the children, with high rates of malnutrition, skin infections, trachoma which leads to blindness, and a lot of water borne disease. Together with the traditional healers and grandmothers we started primary health programmes in 368 homesteads and were concerned about the hundreds of underweight newborn infants.

There was a custom of the mother not eating to allow for an easy delivery, ensuring that the baby would not be too big. Maasai women are ectomorphic—tall and thin with small pelvises. There was a fear in many traditions that the baby might get trapped during delivery. The British Government funded our first Traditional Birth Attendant Programme and over the following 20 years we would train over 3,000 birth attendants in nomadic communities. The effects of these interventions were measured in longitudinal studies that we began in 1985, establishing baselines that were to indicate great improvements in prevalence and cumulative incidences of a wide range of diseases and their frequency of re-infection. Effective hygiene and sanitation as well as water purification began making an impact within the first six months.

From 1984, the head of the Mater, one of Nairobi's leading hospitals, Mary Lavell, was coming with us into the Interior. Mary had been in Africa since 1964 and was a midwife and matron, as well as an expert on breastfeeding. We would often bring her acute paediatric patients and children needing surgery. We would always arrive unannounced, covered in dust, with a young mother and child. There was always a bed, always a welcome, always a solution.

Mary had an easy, calm way about her and gave the best possible help to the child. Every mother was treated like a long lost sister, with a gentleness and warmth and smile that came from a bottomless well of goodness. Mary would often be seen bouncing around the bush along the Tanzanian border, guiding our health team, training young nurses and sharing an experience you can't learn easily. I was once very ill with a fever and was anaemic. Paul Cunningham and Tom Hogan went down to the bush past Magadi, close to Tanzania, and they brought me to the Mater hospital. For three weeks Mary nursed me back to health with a delicious sense of humour in which everything was a pleasure, everything was effortless, nothing was a bother. If you are going to do anything for anyone, anywhere, anytime, it should be done the way Mary does it—with a smile on your face and a pleasure in the doing.

With everything in me I believe that the only path we have to joy is the way of serving each other without looking for anything in return. If there is anything sacred it rests in these three truths:

1. All that is worth being, is selfless love
2. All that is sacred and worth dying for is within love
3. Everything worth dying for is in the essence of love

Every now and then we need to look in the mirror and write from our living breath what it is we live by, what is it that we hold as our creed.

If I was to die this day, what is it in my life that would define me? What is it above all else that has determined my 'me', my actions, my name?

By 1987 I had been living in the bush with the Samburu and the Maasai at such a level of immersion that I often dreamt in Samburu. In time I had become a little odd. In fact, very odd.

In my life I have met many people; some great, some cruel. Some loved me, a few, very few hated me with all their being. They were thankfully eclipsed by the extraordinary love I have been given in my life. Like all men I am full of frailty, failure and brokenness. I am not a brave man, nor do I have riches or material success. Recently my bank closed my account because I always owed them money and my credit card was withdrawn. But I have still managed to spend millions of dollars every year doing what I love above all else, living this dream, and creating tomorrows, and that is more important than anything else.

***

Jean Vanier had once warned that 'community begins in mystery and ends in administration.' Leaders move away from people and into paper. It was so easy to lose contact with the people unless we lived among them, and this was something Professor James McCormick understood profoundly. He came to evaluate our community health projects in 1989. James spent a long time in the bush, working on the mobile clinics, and in the villages among the nomads. One of the many positive ideas he offered was the idea that we might start actually paying those who worked with us. It was something that had never occurred to us and so we started paying something to our full time team. James and his wife, Biddy, had experience in India and I had done my Masters degree in Community Health in Trinity College under him in 1988.

My thesis had been on the beliefs, attitudes and understanding of the Maasai about diarrhoea. It was an important study about something that killed so many of the children these people loved. Diarrhoea is so easily prevented, yet it was killing millions of young children every year. The Maasai have a highly evolved understanding and insight into the different types of diarrhoea. James McCormick shared my concern and excitement at describing what the ancient Maasai understood already about the causes of diarrhoea.

Over the years the programmes we ran bore fruit and in time we saw lasting changes among the communities. This was, I believe, because everything we did was in the tribal dialects, everything was done according to the culture and the values of the people. The decisions, planning, and what was needed came from the grandmothers and the elders—it was theirs. The tribes have survived for centuries in conditions hard to imagine. They have a lot of wisdom and experience. The more you live among the Samburu or the Maasai the more you develop a deep, enduring respect for a world not better than ours, but very different from ours.

***

The subject of a forthcoming book is Global Poverty and the Corruption of International Aid. This reflection is not a discussion on the dangerous shifts in world priorities or responses to poverty. It is important in sharing this journey, however, to say something about the context of my adventure in a rapidly changing environment. There are currents that affect us all. We are, I believe, a part of each other and our lives are not lived in isolation. We might be social animals but we are also cultural, political, economic creatures and are a part of the global dynamic, if only in the brief passing of our moment here.

What we do exists in the context of the world around us. Just as my life was stained and coloured by my childhood, so too was it confronted with the broader context of Africa in the world. I was European, living in an Africa torn by conflict, undergoing traumatic transitions across 40 of its countries. The unrest, civil wars, crumbling apartheid, genocide, and decline of foreign investment, were altering how the world related to Africa. Africa had most of the world's poor and remains the world's most distressed region. My journey could never be blinkered, limited to the nomadic villages we worked in. I could not close my eyes in the bubble of inspiring friends and exciting projects. I knew one thing with absolute certainty: this was not the Garden of Eden, this was a continent in crisis.

Like John O'Shea of Goal, Bob Geldof, Willie Brandt and Nelson Mandela, I had shared deep concerns for many years about the hypocrisy of international aid. While the charities on the ground were struggling to raise pennies, governments were wasting billions. Western governments were using money politically and badly, while Third World governments were stealing it off their own people. It was not until the end of the Cold War that the Europeans and Americans suddenly decided they did not need petty dictators any longer and advocated transparency and accountability (only not for themselves). For decades the Bokassas and Idi Amins had been supported, and oppressive regimes, including that of Saddam Hussein, had received military resources. In a new wave of moral integrity, Western governments moved now towards governance and fair play. While Scandinavian and EU countries campaigned for democracy, their companies extended arms trading. There were two truths—ours and theirs. Since the millennium, the gap between 'them' and 'us' has widened more than ever as paranoia, security, political fundamentalism and the politics of fear slowly gain pace.

The world of international development has always been steeped in corruption and vested interests. Many people quite rightly look at the last 50 years of aid to Africa and wonder why it has been such a litany of failed efforts. We are, in the words of Marcus Aurelius, 174AD, 'too much accustomed to attribute to a single cause that which is the product of several, and the majority of our controversies come from that.' So too with poverty.

The reasons for this are complex and shouldn't be the subject of these reflections, but they are too important to ignore. Some of the problems are unavoidable as they have stained Africa so deeply. The 53 countries have some 900 million people, and 700 million of these are in the Sub-Sahara. The World Bank points out that the six richest people are richer than the 600 million poorest and the 250 richest people own more than the poorest 2.5 billion. To bring that down to us; if I am earning £15,000 a year, I will be twice as rich as 180 Maasai people in a homestead.

The average age in Africa is 17, the average age in Western Europe is 32. Add to this the fact that Sub-Saharan Africa has over 60% of the world's burden of preventable disease, an economy smaller than Libya, and is getting poorer. It is crippled with debt and suffocated by dishonesty. Global development is big business. While fast food, cosmetics, pet food and military spending are all higher, the misery industry is still a multi-billion dollar growth area. There are some 40 international agencies, mostly American, that account for 80% of the world's charity expenditure in Africa. The other 20% is spread between another estimated 65,000 charities and organisations.

When I first came to Africa in 1979 there were over a billion people in the world living in extreme and absolute poverty. In 2006 over half of mankind, that's *over three billion people*, live on less than £1 a day. The GDP of the world's poorest 48 countries is less than the wealth of the three richest people in the world.

***

The problems facing Africa were, and are overwhelming. The scale of the countless emergencies was eclipsed by both inertia in the West and paralysing corruption in Africa itself. In our world the richest 20% of the people consume 81% of global resources and that's rising, so it is going to be difficult to distribute diminishing resources fairly when our society is based on consuming more, but only if you can afford it. The poorest countries in the world combined have less than 1% of the world's external trade.

If we look at world spending priorities, there is an interesting pattern. In 1998, military expenditure was $780 billion, pet food in the US and Europe $17 billion, while perfume expenditure was $12 billion. Ice cream in Europe was $11 billion and cosmetics in the USA, $8 billion.

In the same year, global expenditure on education for all was $6 billion, water and sanitation $9 billion, and reproductive health $12 billion, with basic health and nutrition $13 billion. These gaps have become voids. Of those budgets a large proportion is consumed by management, planning, and consultancies that often absorb whole budgets. One of the reasons there are so many failed development programmes in Africa is to do with reality. So much money is wasted in Africa and so many resources are absorbed by the Lords of Poverty. The reality of many Western donors is locked in log frames and concepts that were born in Washington, delivered on computers. This is nothing new:

> 'The white people, who are trying to make us over into their image, they want us to be what they call "assimilated," bringing the Indians into the mainstream and destroying our own way of life and our own cultural patterns. They believe we should be contented like those whose concept of happiness is materialistic and greedy, which is very different from our way. We want freedom from the white man rather than to be integrated. We don't want any part of the establishment, we want to be free to raise our children in our religion, in our ways, to be able to hunt and fish and live in peace. We don't want power, we don't want to be congressmen, or bankers . . . we want to be ourselves. We want to have our heritage, because we are the owners of this land and because we belong here. The white man says, there is freedom and justice for all. We have had "freedom and justice", and that is why we have been almost exterminated. We shall not forget this.'
>
> *- From the 1927 Grand Council of American Indians*

The plans are created by experts and implemented by managers, evaluated by well paid consultants. There are 400,000 foreign experts advising in Africa. There are also half a million professional Africans who have emigrated since 1990. The tides are going in the wrong direction. The problem comes when a Western mindset encounters other people. There is rarely any room for them to grasp or comprehend the possibility of looking at something in another way.

The study of looking at ways we understand is called epistemology. This gives us our map, our thinking software. All too often in Africa donors arrive, often only meeting each other and English speaking leaders. They determine strategies, sign off on policies and then complain when the programmes fail completely.

USAID is the largest single donor in the world and unashamedly says it provides aid in the furtherance of American policies and American interests. Over two thirds of what it spends is in administration before the money even reaches Africa. Much of the rest is eaten up in a surreal internal self-absorption that has nothing to do with Africans, the poor, results or priorities. Multi-lateral donors are unapologetic in publicising these overheads, insisting it is accountability, an accountability that would bankrupt a commercial enterprise. The system of evaluation evaluates management processes by counting things rather than understanding how things change. This is the introspection of power and the delusion that has seen Africa grow poorer. There are many famous examples of the billions wasted and the obscene overheads of these large organisations. The misery industry is about money: it is a $200 billion profit making conglomerate, the overseers paid in six figures, flying first class, staying in five star hotels on hardship allowance. One has only to visit Rio, New Delhi, Lagos, Lilongwe or Nairobi to see how these people exploit the poor. There is no point increasing development resources until the systems that deliver them are transparent and open.

When I was in Turkana, the Norwegians decided to give a fishing project to the region, so they brought a fishing vessel a thousand miles across East Africa, assembled it, and created a fish processing plant. NORAD, the government aid agency, had brought in experts from Norway. No one actually bothered to ask the Turkana if they wanted to fish or what they believed about fish. The Turkana did not want the fish processing plant and were not involved in any of the planning or discussions. No one asked about their legends or their culture, they just decided to help. It was a classic example of the best of intentions costing millions of dollars. The rusting wreck can still be seen on the shores of Lake Turkana, never used, a monument to misguided good intentions and the question of 'whose reality counts?'.

The British Government donated £3 million to Malawi relief projects in 2005. Of that cash, £586,423 was spent on hotels for a US consultancy agency, the National Democratic Institute. Another £126,062 was allegedly spent on meals.

One project funded by the British Government flew in pens and notebooks from Washington, instead of buying them locally. All money given by the United States has to be spent on US firms. The project involved spending money on setting up parliamentary committees to scrutinise the work of the Malawi Government—most of the money was spent on sending in US experts on democracy and entertaining and holding meetings with Malawian MPs in hotels. A decade ago, 10% of the British aid budget was being spent on consultants. That's now down to 5%, so at least it is being reduced. This type of corruption is less obvious than the excesses of the powerful in the poor world. From Bokassa and Idi Amin to Mugabe and Mengistu, the poor have been feudalised and abused. From Siad Bare to Marcos to apartheid and religious persecution, so much has been done in the name of the people. When I first went to Uganda, I remember millions of dollars being spent on government limousines while the northern pastoralists starved. I was working on a project in India once and went to see a government official who signed a letter on his marble desk with a gold Monte Blanc pen and asked me to give him a laptop for his son.

Once we were sent 12 microscopes so that district hospitals could examine blood slides. The post office not only wanted storage charges for the days we had taken to arrive from the desert, they wanted one of the microscopes as well. We refused and sent all the microscopes to Tanzania instead. The Irish Government intervened directly when a vehicle they had bought for child survival was about to be sold off and bought by a politician instead of reaching the poor.

Many African leaders, most recently Desmond Tutu, challenged other countries to rethink the way they use aid and allocate resources. Many across the poor world have shared the same conviction that the donors themselves need to be educated, the colonialism of 'we know best' and 'we will guide you' needs to be replaced with an honest visible equality where decisions are made in the open, not behind gilded hotel doors. Western leaders have been talking about the uncontrolled corruption in Africa while plundering its resources. They have demanded local capacity but are responsible for the draining of skilled professionals in countries desperate for health services

In 2004, 21% of trained nurses qualified in Kenya were recruited by companies from Western countries. At the same time as demanding health programmes are sustainable in areas of extreme poverty, we must ask which of our own health care systems is sustainable.

We can all react to these and a thousand other examples by becoming frustrated or overwhelmed. It is easy to become disillusioned or drained by the perpetual tidal waves of ineptitude that have extinguished so many opportunities and hopes.

***

Corruption has many faces and even more masks. What often passes as community participation can be manipulation, as trapped in dogma as old religions. Community participation can easily become my empowering a community to be so liberated and enlightened that it actually arrived at the right conclusion. The right conclusion might be that condoms are indeed a sin, or that they are giving me choice, or whatever my manifesto might be. The disturbing trend is the same, that whoever is doing the survey usually finds out exactly what they need to find out to ensure the next pay cheque. Sadly some people become negative or cynical when encountering human frailty. Others become void or hardened. It is unhealthy to close one's eyes to the heaving of life around us, and as the world comes crashing through our perceptions, unless we are awake and learning, we will be drowned and broken by it.

***

There was an American priest who had come to Africa to spend a year in Tanzania. He visited Githunguri. He had been in the Korean War and then served in Vietnam, seeing the darkest side of men at their worst; afraid, heavily armed, and angry. These things had shaped him. One evening he arrived in the Holy Family Cathedral, run by Holy Ghost fathers, and he arrived in bits. Fr Brendan O'Brien spoke Kikuyu well and handed the weary visitor a stiff Jameson whiskey. This man had been through wars, a career listening to every failure men can share. Jay, the American priest, told his story to old ears, to men who had lived long in an old continent and grown wise.

He had arrived in Nairobi the previous day. His first port of call was to see Cardinal Otunga. Having seen the Cardinal he took a bus from Westlands to the city—about a ten minute journey. He put his hand in to his back pocket to get the fare, to discover that his wallet had been stolen. A state of shock set in! Here he was in a city where he knew nobody. He had now lost his passport, his traveller's cheques, his loose money and several letters of introduction to people in Kenya and Tanzania. Brendan tried to reassure him that all would be well. He brought him to the American Embassy, which was nearby, since blown up. We explained his problem to an official. He took him in hand and set about reissuing new documents, contacting the bank, and so on. It would all be okay, but what a way to start his year in the Third World! The thing was that Brendan made him see that he had just gained a valuable experience, far more valuable than anything he had lost. He had been placed in a frightening situation but realised that with a calm resolve, things could be done and problems could be fixed.

As Brendan often said, the first thing to remember about advice is that no one ever takes it. Both Paul and Brendan need a separate book because the adventures and times we shared together brought so much energy, life and wonder that they are, if nothing else, worth sharing for their magic. Brendan had worked long in slums and ghettos and I once asked him what he thought was the most important thing worth living for. He is one of those men truly worth learning from and one who says much with few words, always gentle, always calm.

His answer was, I think, the purest undiluted sense I ever heard. 'Forgiveness . . . It's really just that . . . The power over everyone you meet to forgive them everything they do to you, say to you—nothing is as healing as that, it is raw compassion. Forgiveness only lives in light. It is the child of love and its breath is acceptance.'

Once, winding our way through the mud and open sewers of a ghetto in the drizzle of Kibera in Nairobi, Brendan was hailed by a tiny old woman who came shuffling barefoot through the dirt. She came to him bent and frail and he talked in her mother's tongue long and gently in the rain. He talked with delight, his eyes shining, unhurried, his world suspended, given to her. I was wet and wanted to get into the little car that was parked far away, but Brendan was listening. I mean he was truly, with his whole self, listening. He took the old woman's hands in both of his and smiled and laughed, but did so as if he had just met his own mother. I was looking at someone genuinely placing himself into the life and energy of another world so far from his own, so fragile yet so accepted, so valued and precious. My agitation and impatience was worsened by the rain and the smell, the dirt and the heat. Then the thought passed my mind that if for a single moment one were on earth to meet God, how would the origin of creation meet you? As a prince, an Adonis, as a lord . . . or as a deaf old woman in the desolation of a slum in some forgotten ghetto? Where would we find Love if not here? Where would greatness be if not here?

I watched from a distance. I felt closer to the presence of God in that moment than if I were gazing on the high altar of the greatest Cathedral resplendent in gothic magnificence.

Brendan helped me wade my way through the flies and mud. And as we sat in the car he showed me a little treasure. In the palm of his hand was a wet clump of paper. He teased it open and the paper was warm, gripped by the old woman as she had followed us. There in his wet hand it was, shining and tiny. It was a penny the old woman had given to Fr Brendan to help the poor.

***

ICROSS supported many little projects, giving small grants to communities in India, Uganda, and Ethiopia, as well as Tanzania and Kenya. ICROSS had always operated on very small budgets raised by friends from their friends. Occasional newspaper articles helped greatly and by 1993 we were raising £500,000 a year.

Our efforts were always very rooted in the communities, bypassing the bureaucracies and going straight to the people who mattered. We set up a board of directors in Kenya; seven people who between them had nearly 200 person-years of experience in Africa. I contributed one year to that total.

Our team set off overland into southern Ethiopia, bringing medical supplies to drought stricken areas. It was a hazardous journey through Marsabit's vast wilderness into the isolated tracts of Sidamo. We headed up the Rift Valley. It was months before Live Aid but already the drought had gripped the people by the throat and was choking every hope from them. Women dug in empty river beds for a drop of water, and their tunnels often collapsed, burying them. Children searched for berries and roots, the animals were dead and the old never left their huts. As we turned the dust track through a small gorge early one morning, the sun was blinding and hot dust and sand filled the dry air, and there was nothing but white rock. A loud bang echoed. At the same moment the driver lost control, and we swerved before hitting a large rock slab sideways with a vibrating thud, seeing nothing through the dust.

Before we knew where we were we saw rifles inches away from the windows, pointing at us. Most of the supplies had been hurled off the roof and had scattered behind us after they had shot out our tyres. These men were as afraid as we were and shouted at us in their language, their eyes wide, nervously chewing mirrah stems, a stimulant common in the pastoral tribes. I wondered if Leadisimo would try to do anything, but he had measured the situation and judged wisely. We were taken out of the car and then two of the young men who looked gaunt began throwing everything they could find out onto the dust. Maps, cameras, sunglasses, sleeping bags, torches, all ended up on the ground. Many things were being broken simply from being thrown onto stone but we were still too numb to do anything about it. We were not touched and as soon as they had descended into our world they left carrying what they could. It could have been a lot worse. The only injury was my sunburnt neck, which really stung. We gathered the boxes of medicine, most of which were still okay, and drove back to where we came from, with no tyres, just the wheel rims. The three hour journey took the day and Leadisimo was full of wonderful stories, always calm. The police told us that two people had been shot dead on the same road the previous week. We took a long road in a convoy two weeks later. It took that long to get more tyres, but the land rover never recovered, snaking its way, crablike, despite the best rural mechanics.

***

Our long relationship with the Royal College of Surgeons in Ireland started with Dr Joe Barnes who lectured in tropical medicine, as did Robbie McCabe. Kevin Cahill was the Professor of Tropical Medicine. He was one of the greatest living authorities on tropical disease and cases were referred to him from all over the world. He was John Paul II's physician after he was shot and had treated President Reagan. He had written over 30 books and received honorary Doctorates from 23 universities. He knew Somalia and had influenced clinical tropical medicine for generations of doctors, and was to be one of the great influences on my work.

Kevin Cahill had been in the swamps of the southern Sudan. He had treated tropical disease for decades and he had pioneered new ways of understanding tropical health. He was from the Bronx, and to this day knows more about tropical medicine than any living physician. He opened doors where there were none. Kevin Cahill had become a legend before I met him and his passion and genius changed the understanding of the United States in relation to tropical disease.

Kevin hoped that we 'can make some sense of the world; you can help direct the rushing current of events which we cannot stop; you can discern a pattern amid confusing multiplicity. Hopefully you might do the job better than we have, trying to predict and avoid problems rather than merely deal with them after they explode. I do not mean to advocate a simplistic view of life. I know as well, and maybe better than most, that certainty is a very rare commodity in the larder of human understanding.' This gentle and humble physician worked in 65 countries in his long life, full of compassion. He wrote many books, each about ways to heal. He also wrote these words:

'The temptation may be strong to remain quiet and avoid the fray, to seek security in anonymity, to believe that the individual can have little impact on the multiple systems that affect our lives. Each generation deludes itself by thinking that the demands imposed on it are more rigorous than what its predecessors had to bear; that the problems are more insoluble now than then; that it is suffering a complexity in human life never before encountered. And commencement speakers often encourage this delusion by sending their young listeners off with the charge to resolve the problems that their fathers created.

All of this somehow does not ring true to experience; it is too naive a view of the world. It denies the continuity of human life. People have always needed to overcome the prejudices of the past. Right never triumphed spontaneously over wrong. Integrity has always been maintained only through acts of courage. Compassion has never been worth a damn unless it manifested itself in specific acts of love.'

Kevin Cahill spent his life really changing the world, making it a genuinely better place. This is something we should all try to do. He wrote in 2005, 'We simply cannot afford to allow our dreams to remain mere rhetoric. We must make concrete efforts to try to beat at least some of our swords into ploughshares, to redirect some of the vast resources devoted to the military-industrial complex to those not inconsequential stains on civilization that are called humanitarian crises. Think of refugee camps, tens of millions of displaced persons today—not a possibility but a terrible reality—and, in an ever shrinking world, those once distant problems are our problems, those hell holes are the certain breeding ground for future terrorists. No one has yet devised standardised methods, or satisfactory vehicles, to integrate the ideals and experiences of the university with the anger and frustration of the ignorant, oppressed and ill masses of this world. But their dreams and demands are real, and they will not be stilled, and cannot be crushed.

'Think about this analogy. Even before I had a degree in engineering I was fascinated by the concept of a bridge, a blend of poetry and practicality. By appreciating—and harnessing—tensions and forces, man could span abysses, link separated lands, and create a thing of beauty. But soaring girders and graceful arches must be firmly anchored in a solid foundation, or even minimal loads will cause collapse, destroying both bridge and travellers.'

Professor Kevin Cahill changed the world through action and through his passion and fire. He is the Napoleon of tropical medicine, changing the battlefield, never retreating, always changing the way we think. The imagery of a bridge seems appropriate for those who search for hope in a world where greed and arrogance abound. The prevalence of poverty and political oppression, hunger and disease, prejudice and ignorance can be denied only by the spiritually blind. Somehow the efforts to cross chasms of despair and join the disparate parts of a shattered earth must go beyond the physical. As we fight against the forces of evil that continue to enslave the vast majority of humanity, we need lofty dreams—bridges of hope—to sustain our lonely steps.

Kevin wrote, 'Individual efforts are like a journey into emptiness. Only by forging common bonds can we conquer the gaps that divide us, and only mutual endeavours will build a community where peace, justice, and compassion can thrive. It is in this marriage of disciplines, in the cross-fertilisation of professions, in the new efforts of advanced technology applied to humanitarian action, that I see the best, and maybe the only, remaining framework for survival.'

I believe Kevin is right; this is the future, this synergy of all our resources and passions, this bond united to change the way we see and act.

***

One day I was introduced to Ronan Conroy. Ronan was above all a musician with an encyclopaedic knowledge of classical music. Ronan was kneeling on a carpet, sorting mountains of paper, the space filled with John Tavener's *Mater Christi*, and there were piles of CDs everywhere. I shared the work we were doing in Africa and immediately Ronan agreed to help. It was the beginning of a collaboration that would explore possibilities that would change diarrhoeal prevention. Ronan arrived in Africa soon afterwards—the first of dozens of trips—and was instantly at home. Our first task was to go through the sea of data we had and we began radical new research into belief systems, traditional treatments of disease, and solar disinfection of contaminated drinking water.

Our projects in Africa had expanded and we needed more help to meet new challenges. The Japanese Government helped us set up mobile clinics and the Irish Government supported immunisation and training programmes. By 1990 we had trained over 3,000 health workers and provided grants to over 400 women's groups in nine countries. The British Government built Nyoonyorrie Clinic, which was the headquarters of our health programmes among the Maasai, though I still lived in the traditional manyattas with Sarune, Miriape, Leadisimo and Lemoite. Mirella Riciardi, the Italian photographer, had become famous for a book of photographs called *Vanishing Africa*. Her astounding images captured the grace and energy of Africa and was the first book that portrayed something majestic and powerful. Mirella told me that if you ever want to take a photograph you must ask your soul to touch the spirit of the person you are reflecting. Her profound understanding of beauty captured feelings and dynamics quite unlike anything before.

In 1984, our ICROSS groups organised a small lecture tour to America in a bid to try and raise support, and I made my way to New York. I had been writing articles for *The Lancet* and had an audience waiting for me. Having come from the Northern Deserts I found Nairobi airport big and noisy. It was cold in America but the people's hearts were warm and there was kindness in places where you would least expect to find it. I remember a large, tattooed youth handing me $20 to take back to Africa from him and his buddy. Every day was filled with examples of goodness. It was not about fund raising, but it was about being connected.

There was a deep sense of bonding, of people sharing their stories, their own journeys and worlds. Our little committee in New York was made up of a wonderful diversity. We had the Mayor of Southampton and we had Ann the gentle widow of a great American artist. We had a hospital floor cleaner and a Shinnecock Indian chief. He understood deeply the struggle of the African peoples and told me, 'When we Indians kill meat, we eat it all up. When we dig roots, we make little holes. When we build houses, we make little holes. When we burn grass for grasshoppers, we don't ruin things. We shake down acorns and pine nuts. We don't chop down the trees. We only use dead wood. But the white people plough up the ground, pull down the trees, kill everything . . . the white people pay no attention. How can the spirit of the earth like the white man? . . . everywhere the white man has touched it, it is sore.'

A local doctor, Ken Cairns, brought this group together from every walk of life and as was the hallmark of ICROSS, it was a group, above all, of close friends. We had Sarah Larkin Loening in her late nineties, who was in charge of the mailing list, and Norman Jaffe, a New York architect who was to fund many of our innovative projects in Africa.

The Hamptons were beautiful, with amazing beaches and stunning mansions. Over several years, this dynamic bunch organised many talks and lectures that raised awareness and support for our efforts. Sometimes the contrast between my home in Africa and the wealth of New York was challenging and yet such comparisons are never fruitful, just frustrating. I learnt that the secret was simply to embrace whatever people I was with as openly as possible, whether Maasai on the East African plains or friends in a

Dublin pub. It is important to accept people wherever they are and integrate, touching their world, their realities and worries. If we can celebrate someone by simply listening to them, where they are now, it is a lot more enriching than standing apart. We do not have to embrace someone's lifestyle to understand it, nor do we need to practise someone's culture to live with them authentically.

New York was a world apart; fast, electric, full of energy, and the culture shock was cushioned by the welcome of people who opened their homes and hearts. I talked in people's kitchens and was welcomed into schools. I brought my slides and pictures and talked to student groups and ladies' clubs. I found then and now that the deepest generosity and understanding came from those who were poor themselves. It was always the people who had known need and experienced loss who understood.

One evening I had spoken to a small congregation in a Baptist church near Columbia University. It was a fabulous experience full of joy and singing, dancing and rejoicing, alien to my European past but strikingly similar to Africa. The church meeting was about thanks and praise with an exuberance and unity you could feel. I spoke of what could be done to help those far away, and talked of broken futures and great hopes. I showed images that could have been the children of any one in the hall, and they were one. It was euphoric and transforming, but life has many twists and turns, and that night I took one of them.

I got lost; a common habit of mine in cities. I got utterly lost and ended up in an area that did not look familiar. I could not see any cabs and looking down between the buildings saw in the distance a busy, well lit street, so I quickened my pace. Suddenly my way was blocked by two young men and without warning I was on the ground bent over. A kick between the legs is something so excruciating and shatters your system, sending it into violent recoil. Every nerve, every atom of concentration implodes as one's body addresses the momentary agony, and there is a white flash as blood vanishes from everywhere for a moment and you stop breathing. There was another kick, but my body was still managing the first one.

The secret of coping in these situations is breath control. We have power over our minds—not outside events. Realise this, and we will find strength. When your senses are re-marshalled into responding to anything traumatic, it is important to control how you breathe. In the time before trembling and the delayed response you can control how your body copes through slow, controlled breathing, concentrating completely on the breath itself, not the injury. I had used this technique in training my body to cool down in places where it was very hot or humid. It is part of a process of mind and body control common in contemplative techniques. It is good to remember to empty the mind and to allow the stillness that lives inside us to possess us. This is something you can do even lying on the sidewalk, and it stills the pain. In a sensation almost like pethadine you can feel the calm possessing your body. This too is a place you put yourself, a gift you give yourself, and it works. The pain ebbed away and in time the bruises did too. They took my bag which had all the slides I used for talks. Everything could be replaced. When you get robbed, it is never about what is taken, but it is the aftermath of the invasion into your being that wounds.

That evening, however, belonged to the celeb-ration and joy of those who had welcomed me. We can only be injured or scarred if we choose to be. We have the power within us to overcome darkness with light. I remembered Marcus Aurelius' words:

'When you arise in the morning, think of what a precious privilege it is to be alive—to breathe, to think, to enjoy, to love, life is what our thoughts make it.'

There are many examples in every day where a single unkind word can spoil a wonderful day or an act of unkindness extinguishes all the grace. It is our choice to focus on the energies that come crashing into us. Stillness and inner quiet is not worth having if it can't survive the surprises of daily life, and a spirituality that can only live apart from the dramas of life is one not worth having.

***

I returned to Africa after a few weeks visiting friends and exploring the wonderful art galleries on show in New York, Chicago and Los Angeles. Many of the mobile clinics happened on foot as a group of us would cross the great plains from village to village. In Kenya and Tanzania our close partnership with the Ministry of Health provided us with nurses, though those who were not of the old tribes never stayed. Walking through the bush we could have been in another century. The warriors carried spears. I carried a camera the first few times and for weeks we trekked, content, taking our time in the villages. In time these mobiles were done by vehicles or motor bike. As the programmes grew I handed them over to those we had trained.

One morning while we were getting ready to trek to the escarpment I collapsed. I was weak and dehydrated. Sometimes the fever typical in malaria comes late and it can affect people in different ways. This time the onset of symptoms came like waves all at once.

My friends made the long trek to the north, all the while carrying me, heading towards the capital. The fever had taken over and I had gone yellow. By the time I reached the Mater Hospital in Nairobi I was very ill and the Head, Sr Mary Lavell, called Fr Paul Cunningham. I received the last rites. I was not expected to last the night and Paul sat with me. The doctors were worried but Paul wasn't. He told me afterwards, 'There's a lot more we have to do first.' Slowly I recovered but I had been very ill. The malaria had wiped me out and I just didn't have the physical energy to trek the bush for many months after that. I returned to Europe in 1985.

***

I was no longer the young man who landed in the Karamoja. I had aged more than my years. I had lost my definition, I was wiry and thin, my face dried by the sun, my hair bleached, my brow wrinkled. There was in me though a raw, undiluted sense of pleasure, a base vibrant delight about everything and a gratitude for being. There was a deliciousness in everything, not in big things but in the smallest. The fabric of our daily world is so amazing, the experience and sensation of every smell, touch, voice, moment, is such a miracle. The funny thing is that we get so caught up doing stuff that we lose contact with the miracle, and how mind blowing it really is.

To rekindle an old hobby, I would occasionally do a bronze sculpture, always of people. I have never really found anything more interesting and challenging than to capture the energy and magic of the human form. These were sometimes life-size but it was not until finishing one private commission in Paris that I met Therese, a French ballet dancer who had come to see the statue.

Therese was the most beautiful, ethereal, delightful girl I had ever met. I had utterly nothing to offer anyone. We bonded deeply and there was a full silence between us that I not experienced before.

Therese was quite unlike anyone else I had encountered. She was stunning and woke within me a splendour, as if a great city suddenly turned on all its lights in a blaze of glory. Therese's form was God showing off. She was grace incarnate, the personification of wonder, and everything to her was an adventure. She was a dancer, and despite my innate shyness, I met her friends and found myself discovering another universe of expression and experience. In spring I flourished and in me a child awoke, playing and exploring with an innocence that was natural. Over the months we grew close, we danced and did all those things I had never known. It was a time to just accept the moment and delight in each other. It was inevitable that Therese would come to Africa. Africa never needs to market itself and speaks its own language to our souls.

It did not take long before Therese was in love with the majesty and beauty she saw. For four years she would be back and forth between her blossoming career and our profound communion. If I was ever to have a child born from intimacy it would be from the tenderness and power within our bond. This was a journey that began in laughter and continues in grace. It is said that happiness is when what you think and say and do are in harmony, but it may be even more basic than this: it is when everything within you flows and it is at one with love, when you become love, and this is perhaps our most enduring desire.

***

In the wonderful adventure of our lives we meet so many extraordinary beings, some so rare, who come into our lives and cast light into us, making even the withered and worn parts of us spring into life again. Such people restore us, make us whole and uplift us. One such being in my journey came into my life unexpectedly, as with all good things.

Sharon Wilkinson was one of those people who held onto life with both hands and danced with it. She had come to Africa as a young nurse with her childhood sweetheart, David. In their 20 years there they had done whatever they could to build futures, train, help, give, learn, cherish. David had rescued orphans from Idi Amin's genocide, not once but three times. He was a gracious man with a twinkle in his eye, a deadly sense of humour and no time for people's bullshit.

Sharon threw amazing parties and her house was crowded with waifs and strays, not least the Maasai, Samburu and me. Sharon was head of Marie Stopes, a charity providing reproductive health care for women. We were doing a lot of family planning as well and shared common passions, not least for art and music. Sharon always gave beautiful presents—she was one of those people who really think very carefully and bring you something so special. She brought Ronan hats from Afghanistan and Nepal, and gave me a 1st century Roman lamp from Palestine and a rare Ethiopian Coptic cross. In many ways Sharon grew to know me better than I knew myself and became a mirror into my real thoughts, challenging my self-construction gently and calling me to be myself.

She always was to be at my side, occasionally bending down to raise me from my knees when I fell. We all need someone in our lives who is able to embrace the whole of us, the all, including the contradictions and paradoxes. Sharon was one of those beacons of light that always helped you find the way home, and looked for opportunities to reach out, created opportunities to give, knocked down walls to fight a cruelty.

Sharon and I crossed India working on different medical projects for the British Government, and we would always try to go by train. It's always an adventure going on a train in India. The people are crammed everywhere, on the corridors, on the roof, all polite, always friendly. The vintage trains crawl along and one has a sense they will grind to a halt never to move again, but eventually you do arrive. Sharon was a First Secretary and I was only a consultant, but we would often be greeted by a delegation who in their enthusiasm would lunge at me with adulation, garlands, handshakes and reverence, Sharon, lost in the crowd of minor dignitaries, would be in stitches giggling. The best bit was when they figured out that the five foot four inch female was in fact the person they had come to flatter. Sharon always arrives everywhere with lots of luggage—usually presents for everyone.

We once shared our experiences in Rwanda. Most are better left unsaid because the human soul is never fed by the bloodiness of frenzied hate and there is little we gain from knowing how children were tortured or disposed of as slowly as possible.

In this conversation both of us cried often, knowing ourselves the importance of those days. It was not the flotillas of children impaled alive or the churches packed with neighbours set ablaze but the deliberate choice to seek out others to violate on such a scale. It was the inaction of the Western world and the failure of good men to speak out. The stories of madness in Burundi and Rwanda echoed Auschwitz and even in the Goma camp Sharon recalled the security forces taking men out of the camp and their screams could be heard all through the night as they were humiliated to their deaths in unspeakable ways. Ghandhi said once of these things: 'When I despair, I remember that all through history the way of truth and love has always won. There have been tyrants and murderers and for a time they seem invincible but in the end, they always fall—think of it, always.'

If you were to add up the total of all evil in the world, gather together all the darkness, all the tears and all the terror in frightened hearts . . . If you were to take this and add it to all the cruelty and anguish, loneliness and suffering and make of it a great mountain; all this would be as a grain of sand compared to the love and goodness, kindness and grace that lives in this world. Even in Rwanda there were so many acts of courage, moments of heroism and dignity. You must not lose faith in humanity. Humanity is an ocean; if a few drops of the ocean are dirty, the ocean does not become dirty.

When we look at the world sometimes, it seems as if so much is going wrong. Indeed it is a wounded, hurting place in need of great change and healing. Our politicians are so far away from integrity and honour that it is easy to grow cynical. But when you see the overwhelming goodness, the power of compassion and the things that can be done with nothing, you see the love that we can give. I have wept with Sharon many times but laughed with her a thousand times more. If there was one who understood this journey it was Sharon, and in her was my other self, a better self, shorter perhaps, cleverer, maybe, but definitely better.

We cannot stand and wait for others to act and the examples I have seen, the heroes quietly toiling away have continued to set me on fire. I remember one old nurse in the jungles of Borneo. Martha worked with lepers and while she was knee deep in need, she never once lost her smile. She had qualities in common with all those who enrich us, a delicious sense of humour, a passion and a flow of energy that came from somewhere greater than ourselves.

We see remarkable people all around us and through them we can become better people, if we only learn from their wisdom. When I thought about all those whom I admired and was moved by, I began to see patterns. There were similar attitudes, identical traits and energies.

They enhanced everyone around them and were focused. They all had goals and moved towards them with patience. They were always pushing the boundaries driven from within. They never gave up. Whatever the odds, they never gave up. They were all good at listening, never preached, just acted. Whether it's a mother looking after her child, Desmond Tutu challenging world leaders, or my primary school teacher, they generate happiness wherever they go because they are channels of some more essential energy, instruments of peace, and in being so radiated, joy. There is far too much misery in the world, too much anxiety, and we need to open ourselves to becoming agents of joy.

There are many ways to bring delight and many ways we become grace. I remember visiting a friend in Dublin. Collie works very hard and he was tired after a long day. He was in the kitchen talking to me about something we have both forgotten. I was watching him as he was with his children. His care and gentleness, his concentration towards their little stories and the attention paid to their news. As a dad he was channelling a quality of listening not as common as it should be. During the course of the evening I saw many unconscious gifts, as Collie simply celebrated with such pleasure the gift of his children. We all see many times little acts of kindness, little gifts of love, yet it is these that we should celebrate. If a life is to be measured, it can be so through the love we have given away.

If we are to heal then it is through our undivided attention in the giving of ourselves. Every gift of love is a miracle, and from our hearts can flow many miracles. That evening in a Dublin kitchen, I saw the beauty of unconditional love as a father celebrated the wonder of his children, by simply delighting in their magic, sharing their world, being present to them.

Of children Kahlil Gibran wrote:

'You may house their bodies but not their souls, for their souls dwell in the house of tomorrow, which you cannot visit, not even in your dreams. You may strive to be like them, but seek not to make them like you. For life goes not backward nor tarries with yesterday. You are the bows from which your children as living arrows are sent forth. The archer sees the mark upon the path of the infinite, and He bends you with His might that His arrows may go swift and far. Let your bending in the archer's hand be for gladness; for even

as he loves the arrow that flies, so He loves also the
bow that is stable.'

There is no greater magic than children and no
greater solution to human suffering than gentleness
and compassion. While this is the cornerstone of so
many traditions, sadly humanity has not lived by these
truths. It is still a world in which 50,000 children die
each day from diseases of poverty, a world in which the
response to such injustice is left to people's charity.

I remember getting out of bed one morning, when
Paul and Lemoite had gone off hunting and the camp
fire was being lit. Thoughts lazily strolled through my
head and I looked up at an eagle soaring high above
me and the vast expanse of African sky. I heard the
laughter of children and the sound in the distance
of my friends playing in the stream. I thought about
everything I had, all the gifts, the pleasure, the love
in my life. I found myself laughing and Sarune came
over wondering why I was crying. Could life be this
fantastic; could one life have so much joy? Then it
began to dawn on me, it was optimal experience all
the time. It is when all the energies of our lives find
balance inside us that we experience such flow, such
integration, unconditional happiness.

CHAPTER SIX

'Happiness is something that exists between us and the world—
the people, the creatures, the lot—not inside us. You can open
yourself to happiness by opening yourself to the world. But
you cannot get it inside you.'
- *Ronan Conroy*

The backbone of our work was always for some
reason women. Whether it was Sr Mary Lavell or
Sharon, most of the real success was through, by, and
with women. Our groups raising funds in Ireland and
New York were almost all dynamic women who all
became close friends. In Africa, a close friend was
Áine Costigan, a health professional specialising in
HIV and in programme delivery. Áine was incapable
of bullshit and talked straight with a formidable
intellect and overwhelming integrity. I met her while
sharing research into AIDS orphans at a Nairobi
University conference, and we instantly connected.
Áine worked in the slums and was indefatigable in
fighting for children's rights and women's health. She
had a passion that knew few bounds and a personal
grace that was enviable.

In Africa, everything that worked was through
women's groups, grandmothers and mothers. Our
water committees were made up of women, the orphan support in the villages consisted of women, and
the carers of the terminally ill were almost all women.
The restructuring of ICROSS was needed to meet
new demands and a growing number of programmes

as well as international consultancies. Sally Mukwana was a Ugandan management specialist. She had done work for the British Government and advised the World Bank, and was involved in restructuring major international corporations.

In 1996, the Board of Directors asked her to evaluate the management capacity of ICROSS and make recommendations to move us forward. In order to make the impact we needed on health in Africa we needed to formalise many of the structures that had grown from the villages and communities. Sally developed reporting systems, management capabilities, and training programmes, professionalised the management teams and brought in a new level of administrative personnel. By 1999 ICROSS had transformed from being a series of grassroots programmes and long term relationships into being a competitive non-governmental organisation with a serious network of support within Africa and overseas.

Sally knew how to approach donors and understood the matrix of power structures; we didn't. Our Board of Directors became interdisciplinary, ensuring governments, international donors, the professions and the various health sciences were represented. Dr Evan Sequeira was the foremost gynaecologist and obstetrician in Kenya and headed the ICROSS surgical teams, becoming a very proactive chairman. The Sikh community was closely involved and supportive, drawn in by Davinder Thethy, a businessman who often donated furniture for classrooms and clinics that we built. Sally introduced this capability in time for several major leaps. Not least, she prepared us for a whole new set of challenges as we tackled the new holocaust; the inevitable spread of AIDS.

When I first went to Africa no one had heard of AIDS. It was years later that Dr Joe Barnes told me how the rare Kaposi's sarcoma was so common in the Biafran camps in Nigeria in the early 1960s.

A *sarcoma* is a horrible cancer that develops in connective tissues such as cartilage, bone, fat, muscle, blood vessels, or fibrous tissues. Dr Moritz Kaposi described it in 1872. This disease typically causes tumours to develop in the tissues below the skin surface, or in the mucous membranes of the mouth, nose, or anus. Now it was common. In the late 1980s we started HIV prevention programmes and we were caring for over 300 young Africans who were very ill. Most of these patients were on the shores of Lake Victoria. There was no treatment and the conditions they lived in were extreme. Across Africa the taboo in talking about sexuality created an environment where it was difficult to change behaviour. Even when our local health teams shared safe sex practices, there was little success. We were not alone across the continent: death rates were rising, life expectancy was falling.

The great advances gained in primary health over 40 years were being lost. In villages across western Kenya we were trying to encourage prevention, but the barriers of culture and custom threw up many obstacles and prevented us from getting our message across properly. We would demonstrate the use of a condom using bananas. When we would return to the homes we would be told that the safe sex system was in use, and there carefully placed above the bed was a banana wearing a condom!

***

We always worked together with other partners and organisations. We had helped create dozens of women's groups and self-help groups, but now they were being decimated by the worsening epidemic. No one really knew where to begin. There was a lot of fear and ignorance and across the globe AIDS became the new leprosy. My friend John Hurt did the voice-over for the TV adverts that shocked people into reality, but this was only the beginning. There was worse to come.

Within two years we were looking after 3,000 patients who were weak from multiple infections. Our programmes reached to Lake Victoria and many of our own staff became sick too. Most of the communities we worked with live in absolute poverty and the most basic facilities did not exist. Mothers lay on the earth, too sick to feed their hungry children, neighbours were afraid of the disease and the diseased, and many people were left uncared for.

I had often been asked to write books. For many years after writing my first book, *All Shall Be Well*, I felt that I had little that needed to be shared. *All Shall Be Well* took its name from the mystic Julian of Norwich, who wrote some beautiful insights into celebrating life. She was one of the first free female thinkers whose radical vision of life touched many. She had very deep insights into love and realised that in every way light will draw everything into light and love will infuse everything with love. *All Shall Be Well* was a meditation written in the 1984–1985 East African famine. It was about everything being made whole and complete and expressed a philosophy of integrated compassion. It advocated radical engagement by us all in the suffering of each other and a rethinking of our idea of 'other'. It suggested a new way of thinking about the

'I' and the 'you', the 'us' and 'they' construction of the world. It was about a world unloved, and the victory of gentleness over cruelty.

In that book I told a story about a little island. On the island there lived two tribes. They had everything they could ever need, so much in fact that they exported their grains to many parts of the world. After many years there came a great famine on one part of the island. On the other side of the mountain the others still prospered and did well. Those who had much sat on their side of the island and had a meeting. They discussed how they might help the others on the far side of the mountain. Some of them said that if they fed the children on the far side of the mountain they would become lazy and dependent. They would not work and they will not want to help themselves. Others said that they were all the same blood and all lived on the same island. 'We are one family, one blood; we breathe the same air and weep the same tears. We are one.' The elders spoke for many days, sharing ideas and planning what should be done.

Eventually the elders decided to go to the coffers of the town hall. With great pomp and ceremony they took some silver coins from one of the smaller gilded caskets. They addressed the people on the benefits of helping those poorer than themselves and everybody clapped and cheered at their generosity. A delegation was sent to the other side of the island, but few had ventured there in such a long time.

When the elders climbed at last to the top of the mountain they neared the viewing point from which they could see the whole island. They looked, and they looked, then they stared at each other in amazement. Before them lay the other half of the island, empty, barren, the grave markers scattered as far as the eye

Right: We need to stand up and say what needs to be said: that it is everybody's duty to help those in need. If we don't change now, our legacy will be that the rich sat back and watched as the rest of the world died.
© *Kai Z Feng*

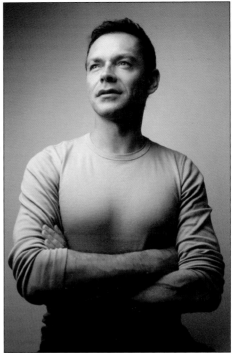

Below: Africa is not a hopeless continent constantly needing our help, but a proud, noble place where people just like us, with the same hopes and dreams, live and love and celebrate their very existence.
© *Author*

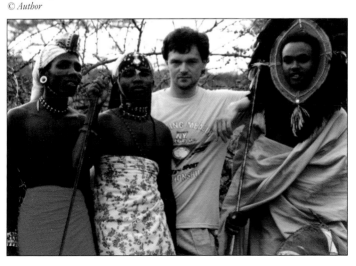

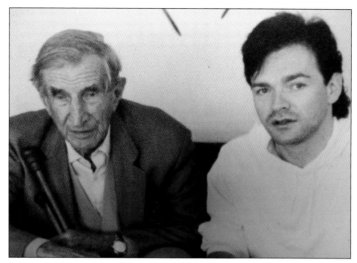

Above: With the late Sir Wilfred Thesiger. He truly was one of the 20th century's greatest explorers and his passion for Africa inspired me. © *Sarune Ole Lenengy*

Below: I have watched ICROSS grow from a small group of dedicated professionals into a multi-disciplinary team of doctors, teachers, journalists, students, carers and more. © *Lemoite Lemako Elmore*

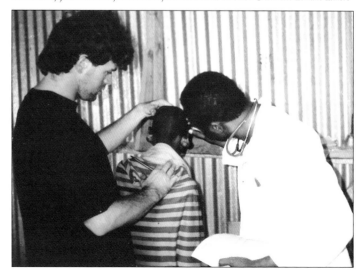

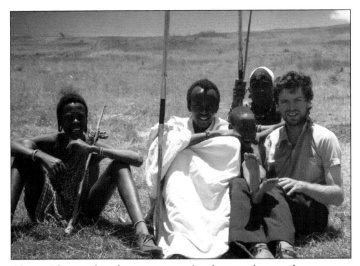

Above: I learnt that the secret was simply to embrace whatever people I was with as openly as possible, whether Maasai on the East African plains or friends in a Dublin pub. © *Gerry McCrudden MBE*

Below: In the beginning we would do mobile clinics on foot. The Japanese Government later donated money to pay for vehicles. © *Miriape Ole Sangaire*

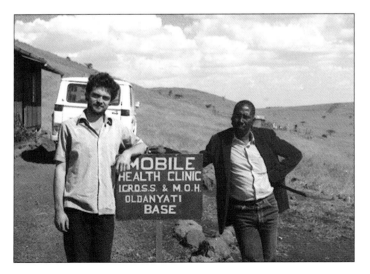

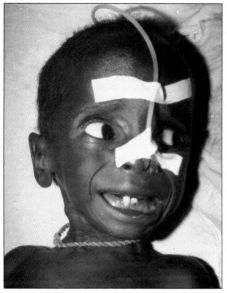

Left: There are huge problems facing children in Africa, with high rates of malnutrition, skin infections, trachoma which leads to blindness, and a lot of water borne disease.
© ICROSS

Below: I noticed the kindness of mothers towards the children of strangers, the gentleness of children towards each other and the dignity of the old who had seen these things before.
© Author

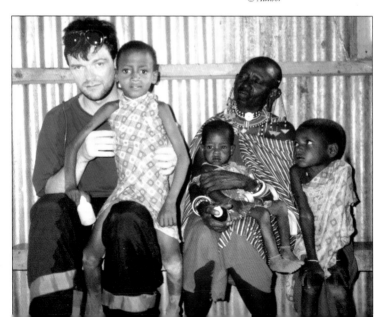

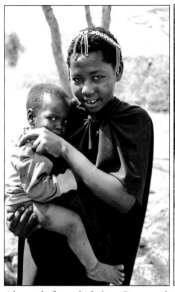
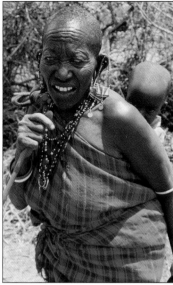

Above left and right: Our work focuses on training mothers in nutrition and hygiene, educating girls, supporting women's groups and preventing HIV. © *Manuel Scrima*

Below: A Manyatta, a simple hut constructed from sticks and cow dung, similar to the one I lived in for many years. © *Manuel Scrima*

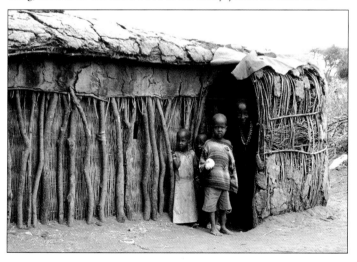

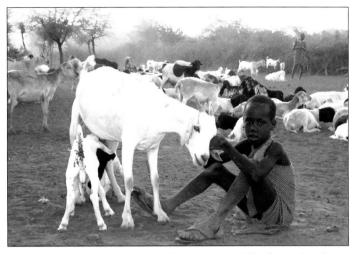

Above: Most tribes we work with have seen 95% of their herds destroyed by drought or famine. © *Manuel Scrima*

Below: The Maasai's connection with their land is always amazing to watch. I never cease to be in awe of their wisdom. © *Manuel Scrima*

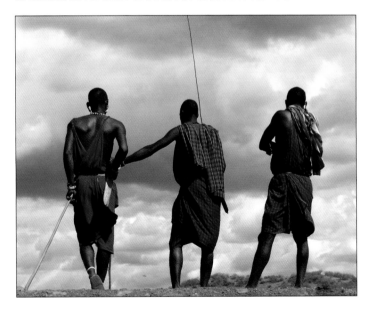

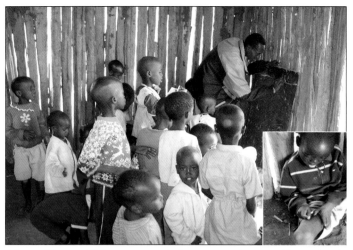

Above: These children averaged about a 90 minute walk to school, which is a small wooden hut with one overworked teacher. They write with twigs on their skin (inset), as there are no books. © *Manuel Scrima*

Below: Many children in Africa have to work full time to help sustain their families. © *Manuel Scrima*

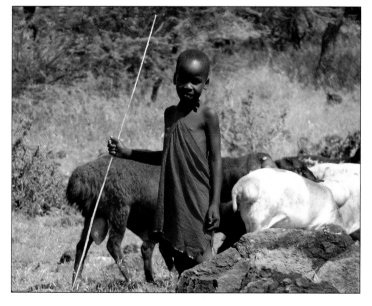

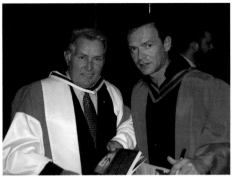

© Courtesy Michael Lee

Left: In April 2006, when I received the Honorary Doctorate in Medicine from the National University of Ireland, I was sure that it was a mistake or just a joke, but it was to be a very personal honour for me. I'm pictured with American actor Martin Sheen.

Right: With Dr Joe Barnes, co-founder and patron of ICROSS. Joe was practising in Africa before the days of charities and NGOs. He was also the first medical doctor working with the medical missionaries and was among the first in the killing fields of Cambodia.

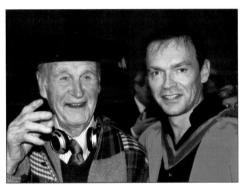

© John Lowes

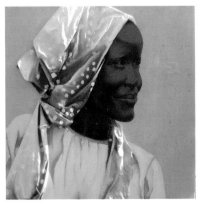

Left: A portrait by artist Peter Homan whose work is featured in an ambitious international exhibition called *Africa Awakes* that offers a new image of the continent.
© Peter Homan

could see. They were too late. They stood on the hilltop a long time in silence, the rain fell upon their faces and there was a rumbling in the heavens. They turned homeward as darkness fell, their eyes full of tears.

***

My own journey was unimportant—what mattered was encouraging others on their own voyage of discovery. Ronan Conroy and I had been researching for many years together. Our collaborations were published internationally in medical journals and both of us were often asked to write pieces on public health and disease in Africa.

I had told the story of Atria, one of the many people we were working with, in the *Journal of the American Medical Association,* in a piece called 'I held him in my arms and wept.' There were over 2,000 responses to that article. A year before his death, 17 year old Atria weighed 98 pounds. He had left his village, he was unwanted and alone, more alone than we could ever imagine. He was afraid and ashamed; the humiliation of the disease eating him made him hide. He trembled and tried to smile but couldn't any more.

In recalling Atria I wrote about his rashes and ulcers, his intestinal worms and the destruction of his body. The reality of being destitute with nowhere to die in dignity, the tears, the fear, is hard to express. I told of Atria's sleepless nights and panic attacks, of how long a few minutes can seem and the sense of powerlessness watching your own body fall away, the humiliation of slow disintegration.

We hear of the tens of millions dying in Africa of AIDS, but the reality is sanitised by statistics and cold data that do not weep or yearn to be held in someone's arms.

Some infections are harder to deal with: a mouth filled with ulcers, an inflamed penis. As the disease progresses so does the nausea, the back pain, the headaches. Muscle cramps always hurt, especially when one has very little muscle. Atria had severe diarrhoea and the dull aches in his stomach became stabbing pains that never stopped. His sight faded, and he grew worse. Atria had stinging, burning pain from urinary tract infections, as his urinary tract was blood red and raw.

Moving his bowels became a nightmare, as his anus had lost its muscular contractility and often got infected. Not eating was better than that. He had no buttocks, not really, just skin stretched over bone, sore to lie on. His joints were hypersensitive. Above all, Atria found it difficult to breathe. His dreadful wheezing-gurgling prevented sleep and he cried because the painkillers no longer worked.

In the months before he died we looked after him as best we could. He was a beautiful young man once, with stunning eyes. He had been a proud, energetic guy, very popular and ambitious, with a sense of fun. Now, most of all he hated that he was leaking and was helpless. He complained that he smelt like he was rotting, and often could not control his bowel movements or urination.

He was too weak to be angry at himself. The slightest knock caused a painful bruise. Atria's weight fell to 84 pounds.

After another few weeks, the boy was drained; his mouth full of thrush, a thick, white fungus over his tongue and gums—and ulcers. He had difficulty swallowing. Breathing was increasingly laboured.

By now, pneumonia had gripped him. Atria's limbs stiffened and his back was covered with ulcers that seeped and bled but did not heal, impossible to manage in a small hut.

We tried to help by controlling pain, managing his distress, reducing fear, creating dignity, reducing multiple infections, reducing cross-infection to others. But the worst thing was loneliness. To die of AIDS in Africa is an intensely humiliating ordeal, slow . . . obscene. We were with him as much as possible. His tear ducts dried up, his hair had fallen out, his bones stuck out. He had no muscle or fat. He had been eaten alive from the inside and there was nothing he could do about it. All of Atria's senses were shutting down. His fingernails and toenails had fallen out. His skin was blistered and scaly, and scabs could not form. The bedsores and ulcers spread, sources of multiple deep infections. Breathing was almost impossible and the slightest movement was slow and full of dread. I gave him water, drop by drop through a straw, but this brought no relief.

I held his frail, stiffened hand. He was cold, he had no tears. I looked into his eyes. I whispered to him, and kissed him. He slowly inhaled, half closed his eyes. He breathed out, very slowly.

Atria's face relaxed, his tormented body sagged . . . I held him in my arms and wept.

***

I cannot describe the fear and emptiness I felt watching such disintegration. The images that flash across my mind are not the data, the plan, the project, but the faces, the faces of those who have had no-one to love them . . . nowhere else to go—outcast, neglected, unwanted.

At the time I wrote these words:

'I feel so inadequate, so useless and unworthy, flawed and pathetic, so utterly overwhelmed. I want to be somewhere else. I am not able for all of this. The horror of the holocaust revolts me. I have sights so unspeakable in my mind. What has humanity done? In my aloneness, in my fear, in my pathetic inadequacy, in my own humanity, despite myself, I fall before the feet of God and cry: Why?

Yet in the end, I find the only thing that matters is to do the best I can.

I leap into the darkness and find myself in a sweltering, disease-ridden place, full of flies and gross smells— and a child is crying. I reach out to gently grasp his small, withered hand, too weak to tremble.

I am here . . . '

Sometimes this is all we can do. It is easy to think of all the things we can't do, but every one of us can do something, and we can do something about everything.

***

Happiness in our lives is always something that just happens. It is a gift, but we are its creators; it is of our own free will that we live it. I remember being in a crowded train once in London and it was cold and raining on a winter morning. Everyone was dressed in dark colours and had their public transport masks on. At the next stop the doors opened and an ice cold gush of air shot through the carriage along with the rain. Next to me appeared a tall, radiant man, beaming and laughing. Fabricio introduced himself, shook my hand, told me how wonderful it was to be in London and how he was enjoying himself so much. He simply shone, and from him bounced a child's pleasure and the people around began to look up and relax a little and smile. No one wears yellow and scarlet quite like a Brazilian, and Fabricio, his Raphaelite hair blowing in the wind, linked me as we left the station, and asked me to show him something. He did not want to see anything in particular, just anything. You don't really meet people like Fabricio, you experience them.

He was one of 11 children and grew up surrounded by love, so he treated everyone the same way he was brought up. He felt mildly amused by those who frowned at him, and could not understand impatience; his top speed, even in the rain, was a slow stroll. Fabricio cried when he called home sometimes and possessed an innocence I had not encountered in the Western world. He now teaches street children how to dance in Sao Paulo and sends me fabulous stories of his adventure.

As Ronan pointed out to me, 'One thing to notice about happiness is that it seems much less personal than some other emotions. When you feel depressed, humiliated, afraid, angry, all these things are unmistakably located within you. But happiness seems accidental, as if it didn't belong to you. People often feel distrustful of happiness, as if it might blow away and they wouldn't be able to call it back. There is no such fear with negative emotions.

'I don't think happiness is an ego emotion. The ego emotions are all to do with possession. Your relationship with your greed or your despair is one of possession. Happiness doesn't seem like something you can possess. Indeed, it scares people how easily it seems it could fly away, or be gone in the morning. I think that this is because happiness is "out there" the way rage is "in there". Happiness is something that exists between us and the world—the people, the creatures, the lot— not inside us. You can open yourself to happiness by opening yourself to the world. But you cannot get it inside you.

'People desperately try to put joy inside them where it will be safe. People tend to abuse the word love, and use it in the sense of "I love hamburgers" or "I love shoes," meaning "I want to consume hamburgers" or "I want to own more and more shoes". This is a forlorn attempt to swallow happiness like a burger or lock it in your wardrobe like a possession. It can never work. Opening yourself to the world isn't just opening yourself to the beautiful sunsets over the ocean or the laughter of children or the smell of freshly baked bread. It's also, as you know, the piss and the shit, the violence, the awfulness. But that's the price you pay —entering into a relationship with the world means action, responsibility. But so does any relationship.

'And perhaps then you will realise that the best guarantee of the permanence of happiness is exactly because it isn't yours, it's everyone's and no-one's. It's out there for us whether we are there or not.

'Truly happy people have learnt to let go of fear, find freedom from the past, and celebrate the present. They are capable of understanding the power of the present. Through this freedom they experience profound enjoyment and delight in the now. Their happiness is not some sheltered delusion of a bright, decent world, it exists in the reality of now with all our brokenness, and it becomes light to that reality.'

For over 25 years there was a man who had worked among the destitute. He was poor himself, and went to school in Bombay. He rose to eminence and became a famous surgeon. He became wealthy and powerful. He lectured around the world and his reputation was revered. He was head of Gynaecology and Obstetrics in a world famous teaching hospital. The same man performed operations every month in the bush. First alone, then bringing together top surgeons, Evan Sequeira went into the most dangerous areas, sometimes saving lives by torch light. Evan brought ICROSS surgical teams deep into the bush and provided the highest standard of surgery in the world to the poorest people on earth. Now a leading doctor involved in international medical research, Dr Sequeira is renowned. Knighted in Portugal, revered in Africa, Evan leads teams of consultants reaching the most remote areas, dealing with the extremes of medicine, not even found in textbooks.

For a decade Evan Sequeira has been the head of ICROSS in Africa and has performed over 2,000 operations in extreme conditions. He never notices that he gives—it is simply his nature.

The bridges of our lives are those people who fill us with joy and grace, those who test us, awaken and challenge us. Just as I was fortunate enough to have so many wonderful influences in my childhood, I am fortunate as an adult to have so many amazing people coming into my life to guide me on my own journey. Atria challenges my humanity, Fabricio my living in the now, Ronan awakens my mind and Evan shows me humility. Our journey is about just this, what we discover along the way, how we grow and become, awaken and celebrate that discovery in each moment. For me the journey is always more and more amazing.

Each time I get out of bed in the morning, from the base of my stomach comes a word . . . wow!

CHAPTER SEVEN

'The world is full of suffering; it is also full of overcoming it.'
- *Helen Keller*

If you want to understand the history of the last century, study Hell: Dante's Hell. Our history, however bloodstained, has another and deeper meaning. It is not the evil and cruelty of history that is significant. It is not by the madness and greed of our time that we will be measured or understood. The world of those who heal and love is united in joy. The world of those who are angry and full of hate is consumed in their own abyss.

If we want to understand ourselves we need to understand how we behave in the face of madness and in a world mutilated by our own insatiable capacity to hurt each other. I cannot realise my full humanity without embracing the brokenness of those who are afraid and hurt—unless I have compassion for them. I must have at least enough compassion to want to ease their suffering. If for some reason I do not spontaneously feel this desire for others, then I must do all in my power to find that compassion within my heart.

The world was changing and as new states emerged, old enmities rose from the past. Hatreds born long ago would rise and tear tomorrow from bright eyed children. Somalia, Bosnia and Rwanda were about to unfold in front of the world, and much of the time we had our eyes closed.

ICROSS had a series of small projects running in Somalia since 1986. Working closely with Italians in Mogadishu and outlying areas, we were supporting water programmes and the development of labs in hospitals. We were able to introduce a small maternal child project and Bare Ali was going to be coordinating it. Before he could apply for a visa he was arrested and deported as a spy. Somalia was in a rapid nose-dive and violence was flaring up in outlying areas. In 1992, responding to the political chaos and humanitarian disaster in Somalia, the United States and other nations had launched peacekeeping operations to create an environment in which help could be delivered to the Somali people. By March 1993, famine had been averted, but the security situation collapsed. On 12 July 1993 a young photographer, Dan Eldon, was beaten to death by a crowd. He loved the Maasai and the Ngong Hills. He was a talented and award winning journalist just launching his international career, with so much promise. He was 23. Somalia was a total failure by any measure, and everything that could go wrong, did go wrong. The international agencies had done their very best, the UN had really tried, but Somalia was too busy tearing itself apart. The UN withdrew in 1995, after suffering significant casualties, and order still had not been restored. There is still no government in Somalia.

At the same time, the Middle East and changes in the emergence of the new countries of Eastern Europe filled the foreign news sections of newspapers. Since 1992, the Bosnia-Herzegovina conflict between the three main ethnic groups—the Serbs, Croats, and

Muslims—resulted in genocides committed by the Serbs against the Muslims in Bosnia, and many more atrocities on both sides. The unfolding lunacy and litany of madness was beamed into our sitting rooms. We saw starved young men in detention camps. They were white, they were European, they were us. I was very impressed with General Lew McKenzie, who commanded the UN peacekeepers in Bosnia and was responsible for bringing stability into a situation that had spun out of control. He kept Sarajevo airport open and ensured relief supplies as the factions tore each other apart. He was later to become the patron of ICROSS in Canada, working with AIDS orphans and very vulnerable children.

It wasn't until May 1994 that Africa returned to the headlines with a vengeance. Between April and June, nearly a million people were murdered in 100 days of frenzied killing. Rwanda had exploded into a fevered genocide that stunned the world. Many people saw the madness coming. Since 1916, when the Belgians had issued identity cards, the Hutu and Tutsi were divided. In 1959, 20,000 died in riots, and nothing was done as divisions mounted in the early 1990s. Despite every warning, the international community did not attempt to avert the tragedy. It was not until hundreds of thousands had been tortured and hacked to death that the international community decided to enter Rwanda. By then the carnage had reached every village. Depending on tribe, a husband would be forced to kill his wife and children, a teacher to pour petrol on a student and set him or her on fire. The stories went from the perverse to the unfathomable, and revulsion was replaced by numbness as sensory overload took over.

I was there to witness the aftermath of some of the worst massacres and acts of barbarity, but what happened in churches and homes, primary school classrooms and peaceful village market places defies understanding and description. We are not equipped with language that can reach that far, in experience or fiction.

The horrific thing is that Rwanda was not a once off situation, and death, in whatever form it took, was a constant shadow over the work of every NGO and charity. Throughout the 1990s, the barrage of human crises and tragedy gradually created an understandable sense of futility in many people. It seemed that whatever our good intentions and best efforts, some parts of the world just could not escape themselves.

Since 1998, over three million people have been killed in the Congo. Since 1983, two million have died in the Sudanese civil war. 70,000 died in the first six months of 1998, many of them starved to death. In Darfur, people have died from lack of water, despite water being close by. Raiders armed by the government slaughtered whole villages. In April 2002, Angola ended a 26 year civil war that saw atrocities every month. Three factions in Liberia destroyed the whole country in a savage and macabre civil war that raged between 1989–1996. There are many more examples. In the midst of this was a collapsed economy in most of Africa, and while resources were invested in armies, there was no infrastructure. Added to this was the growing AIDS crisis, an epidemic that was largely misunderstood.

***

As AIDS began to cause unimaginable suffering among the poor, there were mixed reactions. Many leaders, including the Kenyan President, were in denial. They either did not believe that this disease was ravaging their people or they did not accept the Western agendas and plans of prevention. There was a complex mix of politics, fear, ignorance and stigma, and the result was continental inaction. Only after some ten million Africans had died did most governments start to introduce policies. They were all too often poorly designed and the international organisations, while doing their best, were limited without political support. Senegal, Uganda and South Africa had aggressive prevention programmes reaching from the slums and the prostitutes to the remote market places, but they were the exception to the rule. The Catholic Church in Africa was not helpful with a continued opposition to the use of condoms. In 1993, ICROSS distributed over a million condoms but the efforts of the non-governmental organisations and the Ministry of Health still left many millions of unprotected acts of sexual intercourse.

The politically correct language of the day prevented open discussion about sexual behaviour. HIV was spreading in schools but many African countries were not ready to provide sex education to young teenagers as they felt it would not be culturally acceptable. Cardinal Otunga and the Imam of the Jamia mosque had a burning of sex education materials in 1995 and by 1996 stockpiles of condoms went up in flames. Otunga was not alone. In Africa many conservative and traditional groups as well as political factions had theories about HIV. Many thought it was a Western invention designed to cull Africa's population. Others noted the growth of very well funded Western organisations across the Sub-Sahara, busily trying to keep the population down. Some even suggested there were contraceptives in the school milk. Conspiracy theories grew with waves of disconnected anti-Western feeling. At the time the major donors had reduced international aid substantially, requiring reform. Western governments were demanding transparency, accountability, democracy. When the Berlin Wall came down in 1989, the strategic advantage of African states changed and Western resources often spent to placate and manipulate dictators could now be channelled more usefully.

The United States in particular saw an opportunity to force African governments to reform the un-controlled abuses and corruption that had crippled growth. The reaction was a series of tensions that underpin the uneasy dialogues today. The public in Western countries were tired of the endless stories of corruption and disease. It seemed that no matter what was given to Africa it was either stolen, looted, broken, misused or it failed.

People were tired of the corruption and dishonesty, the fighting, and the greed of dictators, so there was little opposition to shifts in international development priorities. There was a communal turning away from the problem.

I was living mostly in Maasai villages at the time, simply trying to persevere in the face of overwhelming problems, but we were at least trying to make a difference. By the early 1990s our own development projects had become very successful and cost effective. Over three quarters of our work was in Western Kenya. ICROSS in Tanzania had become completely autonomous, run by Job Lusinde, based in Dodoma.

In Tanzania our work focused on training mothers in nutrition and hygiene, educating girls, supporting women's groups and preventing HIV. These prog-rammes were working, but we needed to address the problem of the world's view of Africa; something we are still trying to do to this day.

In the mid-1990s, many of us in ICROSS and other development organisations felt that we should do more to educate the public in Europe about the other Africa, the Africa they never saw. The West only heard of the achievements of dictators and despots, the results of greed and famine. The other 700 million Africans scattered across 12 million square miles were unseen. The caricature of Africa had been formed by reinforcing the imagery to the point that even my friends in London and New York had created stereotypes that governed their thinking. Once I was talking about new hopes for Africa in Paris, when a question came from the audience.

'Why should we waste our tax francs on people who are thieves, live in palaces, oppress their own poor? Does not the work you do help those corrupt officials who fail in their own responsibility? You don't seem angry about this? Maybe you should be . . .'

It was a good question, and one I ask myself on occasion. The answer is that we should not channel anything through governments. We should work through organisations we can hold accountable, because we can't hold other governments accountable. Whether it be Oxfam or ActionAid, CARE or Médecins Sans Frontières, we can choose avenues that can really impact in an area we are interested in. If I decide not to reach out to a child in a slum because the rich politician has a big Mercedes, I punish that child because of the greed of his oppressor. The child becomes a victim of my moral objection. It does not make me angry because I have never seen any goodness come from anger. Anger is a negative energy, a very powerful negative emotion that consumes a lot of inner resource, and all the anger in the world has never yet fed a single child. There are a lot of people ready to get angry and frustrated, annoyed and furious. In my experience, it is not this group of people who make the world a better place.

Against the backdrop of changing global priorities, the international community continued to respond to epidemics and droughts, disasters and tragedies. They did so as they always do, with a short term 'fire brigade' reaction, often fragmented, rarely learning from decades of limited results and poor management.

In part, the problem lay in the lack of institutional memory of even the largest organisations and in part in governmental policies that had no continuity. The agendas of Western governments were driven not by creating effective long term change but by political expediency, profile and pressure groups within their own countries. Project funding evolved in the early 1990s into funding sector development. Most Western governments ploughed overseas aid into African treasuries, much of it never to be seen or accounted for. Billions of dollars were also allocated to the United Nations and other multilateral bodies whose overheads and operating costs were many times higher than private business.

When the Department of Overseas Development in the UK cut the budgets to charities like Oxfam and Save the Children, it channelled even more money into African governments. Although it was well-intentioned, international charities, specialists in public health and development, warned that this money would not reach the poor. It didn't.

Many sources of funding were tied to very narrow criteria. There were funds for HIV and for malaria, for AIDS orphans and for training nurses. Many of these nurses once qualified were recruited by the British, Canadian, American and Australian health services, who were short of nursing staff. The problem with projects that are subject and disease focused is this: you often have money to cure malaria in 1,000 children, but no budget to buy bed nets or prevent malaria. We often had funding to help children orphaned by AIDS but not if they were orphaned from starvation or cholera. The limitations and restrictions entered the theatre of the absurd with the European Union. Due to the scale of corruption within the EU that had changed its name five times during the course of one application process, a strange bureaucracy was developed. We applied in March 1992 for funding to prevent diarrhoea in children. It was a simple programme requested by the community and the Ministry of Health in Kenya. In a single year, for one application, we sent nine copies of a proposal to Brussels. Each copy was over 400 pages. The office in Brussels then moved and the process was repeated, but three months later a third set of nine copies were sent because they had lost the file. During this Beckettian experience there were four different desk officers handling the application.

By December 1993 we were told that the funding category we had applied for had now ended and there was a new process for a different application process in a newly created office. We began again and redid all the applications, sent in all the audited accounts and fresh letters of support, detailed templates were completed and 16 pages of budgets were compiled in Sterling, Euros and Kenyan currency. We sent the heavy box to Brussels, registered. A month later a new desk officer wrote to us asking us to resend the application. After $2,500 and 12 months we decided to do the programme without EU funding. This only cemented my views that in order for aid to work, it had to come through NGOs. We were able to do a lot more work, a lot more good, once we threw off the shackles of centralised bureaucracy. It also underlined the importance for me of personal experience, living with the very people I was trying to help. I knew the urgency needed, because I was there, I saw the suffering before my eyes, and I saw how I could help. A clerk in Brussels could not.

I also felt a much keener sense of the kindness and love that was needed to help those most in need, and I saw the joy and wonder that flowed through those who gave it, and those who received it.

***

Life is not about hiding from the drama and conflict but sailing through it. We find our balance in the depths of friendship, the heights of vision and the pleasure of action. We are made complete by the love we share and the celebration of the little things that fill our days. These miracles and joys are so abundant that they grossly outweigh the dross and minor irritations that are part of life. Inner joy is not about escaping from human suffering but seeing it for what it is and doing something about it without being diminished. It is about an outpouring of energy with both eyes open, aware of the realities and needs. Real happiness, I believe, is something we create and give; it lies in an insatiable discovery of the goodness all around us, and a celebration of life. It is the becoming of ourselves in the midst of everything around us and finding that everything that is essential is within us. It is the ultimate surprise that everything is truly amazing and really sacred, and that in the things that matter in our lives everything can become pure wonder and delight.

CHAPTER EIGHT

'Society is measured by the way it cares for its weakest members; the weak, the old, the children.'
- *Ghandhi*

By 1994 our work in Africa had drawn a lot of interest from others working in the poor world. There was growing interest in our approach. We were not alone; there were experts from around the world working on solutions combating poverty. We were part of exciting initiatives and collaborations sharing cutting edge ideas. We were in touch with groups on every continent and all of our work involved input from the USA, Canada, France, Belgium, the UK, and numerous African and Asian collaborators from many organisations and institutions. We were working with anthropologists, physicists, sociologists, educators, microbiologists, journalists, child psychologists and policy makers. Colleagues came from Asia and the Americas and we were all exploring the boundaries. About the same time, the internet started to become a possibility in Africa. We had a number of offices in towns scattered across Kenya and Tanzania. It became increasingly possible to talk to anyone, everywhere.

My own unsteady steps into cyberspace were guided by Bob, whom I met online, explaining all that was needed. He explained without the jargon or the spiel, just telling me to press that key and then this would happen, and it did. Bob spent hours every week teaching me how to make things work and configuring everything, all through virtual technology. In time I was able to speed around the net (in as far as you can on dial-up in Africa).

I was grateful and invited Bill for a drink some time, to which he replied:

'Can I bring my dad?'

'Urr . . . hmm Bob, how old are you?'

'11,' was the reply.

It turned out that Bob was the son of a famous malaria researcher.

I believed that health was not something that lived in a project. Health programmes were not about disease and illness, they were about beliefs and behaviour. We created a number of innovative approaches in fighting poverty and bad health practice. Most initiatives tend to start off with the disease treatment model of clinical management. Hospitals and health centres follow a Western approach to doctor–patient communication, and the patient, often in long lines, is gradually disempowered and reduced simply by being present in an alien place. In the Western world too, we struggle with the loss of personal identity and power when in hospital. In Africa the gap is far greater. Between 1979 and 1994 we had developed an integrated idea, based on local values, that should be obvious but isn't.

We had always worked through the local values and cultures of the tribes we were with. Our health teams were always from the community and not educated outside to the point that their aspirations changed. The thinking, the cosmology, the idea of how everything works was inherently and deeply their own. The ideas that were shared to improve health belonged to them. Ownership started and finished with the people themselves, so there was no need for branding, labelling, marketing. The planning came not from donors but from the Elders and grandmothers. The dispensaries and clinics were owned by the community and the power and control belonged to the people. It was going to be the way of the people, which was very different than the way of the Western model of change. As the Sioux Chief Sitting Bull said:

'I am a red man. If the Great Spirit had desired me to be a white man he would have made me so in the first place. He put in your heart certain wishes and plans, in my heart he put other and different desires. Each man is good in his sight. It is not necessary for eagles to be crows. We are poor, but we are free. No white man controls our footsteps. If we must die . . . we die defending our rights.'

***

Our lives are not separated by academic classifications or social groupings. We are living in a dynamic of what's around us. There is my inner self, and there is my extended self—the family, sub-clan, clan tribe, related tribe. This is how I relate to the immediate external things and how I relate to the broader world.

I was heavily involved in trying to find cost free solutions to problems that were crippling villages and communities, because realistically, if it had to be paid for, it could not be afforded.

Each year there are nearly a million deaths from neo-natal tetanus; 80% of them in Africa. The Maasai had a lot of infant deaths from tetanus. This was due to the practice of smearing the umbilical stump with a compound including cow dung. Back in 1981 we had started to work with traditional healers and grandmothers, looking at the beliefs and mythology around the custom. We then asked the old men who were the guardians of the tradition to explain the legends about the role of cattle in the Maasai culture.

Everything revolved around the cattle. Thousands of years ago the pastoral peoples of the Nile depended on the herds for everything. Their descendants became the Nuba and the Dinka of the Sudan. The proto-Nilotic tribes moved through Sudan, spreading by the 15th century into Uganda and Kenya and as far as northern Tanzania and Ethiopia. We found out that the cattle in legend came from the water, and so we used this source as an idea. If the ritual prayers over newborn babies used the origin of the cattle and animals, it might be compatible with the custom. We had the legend shared with traditional midwives and the idea of using water and sterile delivery kits explained by the traditional leaders through their own language. We followed the communities and compared thousands of births. We needed to see how the change would make a difference. It was not enough to look at newborn babies for a couple of years; we kept looking for 20 years. In August 2001, we published the largest and longest study of its kind ever done in Africa in *The Lancet*. It showed dramatic long term change in a project that actually cost nothing to do; only time, trust, acceptance and listening.

Together with tribal communities we began developing long term programmes among nomads to see if we could really change the burden of disease that caused so much suffering. The cycles of poverty could only be broken by consistent and continued shifts in behaviour and practice. Some changes would be more challenging than others. Respecting other peoples' reality was the secret, something that foreign governments were historically not good at. The relationship with the Royal College of Surgeons created new possibilities. The visionary perspective of cutting edge researchers allowed us to become innovative in trying to fight poverty.

One of the worst killers in the world is diarrhoea, which wipes out more children than AIDS every year. A main cause of diarrhoea is contaminated water. Over 600 million Africans do not have clean water and for many years we worked to try and improve water in desert and remote areas.

I had diarrhoea many times in the bush, and sometimes it was so bad that dehydration would come on very quickly. Much of Africa has dry heat and you don't notice the evaporation, as you don't sweat the way you do on the tropical coast lines. I remember an old Maasai man running his tongue along my forearm and telling me I had brown urine. He was actually right. What he actually did was lick my sweat to see if it was salty. I had become so dehydrated that I had perspired all the salt in my body and needed electrolytes.

Diarrhoeal disease is very easily prevented and easily treated. We began working with the tribal mothers on ways of reducing the deaths and re-infections.

By 1995 we had adapted a technology known to the ancient Egyptians but for some unknown reason, not used since. We were going to use sunlight to disinfect the contaminated water. After exhaustive laboratory tests and microbiological analysis it was time to put our theories to the test. Most of the water was putrid and dark.

The Maasai were so used to dirty water that when I gave an old man a glass of clear water he thought it did not look right. He bent down, took a pinch of earth and put it in the glass and smiled. We were going to use empty plastic bottles and put the filthy water in the sun. We were going to measure the levels of living bacteria and disease agents after different lengths of time. After this lengthy research had been published by our team we were ready to see if the solar disinfection would actually reduce the amount of infection in children. Before we began seeing if we could reduce the rate of infections, a few of us started using the bottles ourselves, not without some side effects. I once used a bottle of water but did not know it had not been in the sun. I had the most horrific disembowelling diarrhoea for a week.

We were working throughout the mid-1990s on a range of needs identified by local tribes. Our programmes were spreading and by 1996 we had water projects in many western Kenyan villages as well as nomadic areas. Our independent ICROSS team in Tanzania, with the much loved ex-ambassador to China and Kenya, Job Lusinde, introduced and implemented the diarrhoeal prevention programmes and success followed success until solar disinfection became widely known and our control trials, demonstrating sustained changes in the burden of disease, were published internationally. The simple method of exposing infected water to sunlight even worked during a cholera outbreak. Our solar disinfection was so successful that a series of other programmes began around the world and we began advising other initiatives in Asia throughout the 1990s.

One of the real concerns in East Africa is trachoma, a parasite that causes blindness. Six million people worldwide are blind due to trachoma. Trachoma is one of the earliest recorded eye diseases; it was identified by the Egyptians in 2700 B.C. It is the leading cause of blindness worldwide, and affects over 400 million people (primarily in the poorest countries in Africa and Asia). It is preventable with adequate diet, proper sanitation, and education. It causes terrible suffering and is common in children. With symptoms of tearing, photophobia, pain, red swelling of eyelids, and superior keratitis; as it passes through four stages, the conjunctival tissues become follicular, heal, and finally scar. Tear glands and ducts are affected; the upper lid turns inward and the lashes then abrade the cornea; corneal ulceration results, becomes painfully infected, often festering, and ultimately scars. When scarring is extensive, blindness results. Through the discharge from an infected child's eyes, trachoma is passed on by hands, on clothing, or by flies that land on the face of the infected child. Among the pastoral nomads where children are covered in flies, the sheer density of these flies was a key route of transmission.

Together with David Morley, we spent several years developing a zero-cost fly trap that could be used in reducing the fly populations. We tested a wide range of baits ranging from rotted meat to putrefied protein, but we eventually found out that the most attractive smell to flies was early morning children's urine. We went through a lot to find this out. The fly traps proved a great success and we started clinical trials to see if we could make a real impact on the pattern of trachoma. For three years we studied the patterns of fly swarms and their behaviour, as well as monitoring the seasonality of trachoma in patients across a 6,000 square mile area.

Together with an aggressive sanitation and hygiene programme and fast treatment with antibiotics, environmental efforts, and education, a lot can be done, but in areas where tribes live with their herds the flies would be a massive problem. We introduced our fly traps and carefully measured any impact. Our results were shared in 2000 and 2001 at the International Trachoma Meeting of the World Health Organisation in Geneva. Our results were very exciting and we showed real reductions in trachoma, results we continued to build on and publish internationally. Together with the Royal College of Surgeons we published further promising findings and continue to develop new ways of reducing flies and decreasing trachoma.

Another area of concern was child survival. Over half of the world population is malnourished. This means that over 3 billion people will be going to bed hungry tonight. This is a horrific indictment on world leaders at a time when there is no valid reason for such suffering. The combined wealth of the world's 200 richest people hit $1 trillion in 1999; the combined incomes of the 582 million people living in the 43 least developed countries is $146 billion. 50,000 children die each day due to poverty. 50,000 every day. And they die quietly in some of the poorest villages on earth unnoticed, ignored. They are far removed from the scrutiny and the conscience of the world. Being meek and weak in life makes these dying multitudes even more invisible in death. Many of these deaths can be prevented.

In communities with high infant mortality and malnutrition it is important to make children grow properly. David Morley developed a fresh approach to growth monitoring made possible by the development of an entirely new method of weighing through the introduction of the direct recording scale, which has a large visible spring. Our intention was to get mothers weighing their own children. Over the course of a year, about 90% of the mothers weighing their children on a direct recording scale came to understand child growth as shown on a weight-for-age chart. This was very important and created a home based way of keeping an eye on children who were often ill.

Mothers knew why children should be weighed, and could recognise a normal and an abnormal growth chart. Among a similar group of mothers whose children were weighed on a dial scale by a community health worker, there was little change in their understanding of growth monitoring.

Over a two year period, another showed that a high proportion of the grandmothers, who are the decision makers, as well as the older girls, who are the future mothers, in the families gained a similar knowledge of the meaning of the growth curve. Even half of the fathers and older boys, who are not usually concerned with small children, gained a reasonable understanding of the growth curve.

***

Ronan had introduced me to the writings of Primo Levi. His dignity and courage in the face of degradation and humiliation in the Nazi concentration camps serve as a beacon to all humanity. He endured the nightmare of the annihilation of all he loved, and within himself still lived with grace and gentleness, compassion, and the core of his own humanity.

Ronan was visiting several times a year and every visit to the bush would bring fresh ideas, new authors, new subjects, and dozens of recordings of new music. I had many visitors from different parts of the world who came to see our work. I asked each of them to bring a couple of their favourite books and a little of the music that touched them so that over the years I heard ethnic music from every part of the world, and became exposed to the literature of Brazil and Cuba, Peru and Japan. We had Lithuanians singing folk songs and Buddhists chanting. A poet from Mongolia used to sit by the camp fire with a strange melodious hum and French nurses would recite love poetry. The effect of welcoming the stranger is to enrich your home. There is a saying in Samburu: 'May your home have many gates, and may no-one want to leave.' The wealth of culture, language, tradition and new exciting ideas flooded my life and the lives of everybody involved in the programmes, and we eventually had so many visitors to Africa that we built a small guest house with room for six people.

It has never been empty since 1994. It is a policy of sharing, listening, learning and exchanging that has deeply enriched everyone. For many years we lived only in Maasai homes, where the welcome was the same for me as for a long lost child. One of the most powerful, enduring memories people take away from Africa is the way in which everything is shared, everything is given. People are not attached to stuff in the way we are. They are not conditioned to collect things or possess things in the way we have been conditioned.

I have always believed that the only way to live with people is to share and redefine 'belong'. I have often been in homes where no-one has ever owned a pair of shoes and there was one small tin cup shared by the family. In such homes there is always joy. There is nothing noble or enviable about extreme poverty but there is something we often lose in our pursuit of possessions. I once made a list of the happiest people I knew. It was an easy list to write. I was always fascinated by happiness as it seems to thrive in the most unexpected places. My list included 16 nomads, five old missionaries, five people who lived in another world after living delightful celebrations here. Then there was Sharon and myself. No-one is always happy, but I always sensed I had way more than a fair share. I was deeply loved, surrounded by those who accepted me. I delighted in every waking moment and woke up every day thrilled to be where I was. I almost felt I was missing something rather basic.

I had never felt the distress or depression some friends went through, and stress was alien. There were only two things I found difficult in my life. Both in different ways were absences. I always lacked the resources to implement our programmes properly, and ICROSS would probably always be struggling like the rest of Africa. It was often hand to mouth. For the first 20 years we had an empty bank account at the end of the month.

The second absence in my life was a personal relationship. Having spent most of my life celibate and centred on the contemplative life, I did wonder about the wisdom in monastic traditions of not sharing our magic with another. As I grew older I sensed this more profoundly. I had loved Therese with all my heart but encouraged her to focus her energies in Paris where she flourished and grew perfectly. The love between us grew richer like old wine and her spirit awoke every time she came to Africa. Anything in any way beautiful, such as her, derives its beauty from itself and asks nothing beyond itself. Praise is no part of it, for nothing is made worse or better by praise. After six years of raw pleasure I introduced her to a close friend, also a dancer, from Rome. I knew them both well and nurtured a flickering flame both tried to extinguish due to a love of me. In the fullness of time they became lovers and the magnificent flower of our love grew into another joy and I became the godfather to their son, whom they called Michael Elmore Fabricio after me.

Bright darkness came into my life after a series of losses. Babu Achieng was a magistrate who fought crime and corruption. He lived for the truth and for his family. He worked closely with ICROSS and was on the Board of Directors. He freed the innocent and set free widows who had land stolen by greedy developers. He protected orphans and challenged corrupt officials. For a time Kenya tottered on the brink of civil war with growing anger at wide scale corruption. The old regime was clinging onto power but it was sliding from their grasp. Babu released political detainees and one morning as he went to buy ice cream with his youngest daughter he was shot dead. Ronan put his favourite scarf across Babu's exploded neck in the coffin.

At the same time Fr Paul Cunningham who had walked with me so far had finally died in Dublin. He had only ever brought joy into this world. In all my years with Paul I had only danced and laughed and been awestruck by him. This Holy Ghost missionary had given everything he ever had to everyone he met. When he left Kenya for the last time he carried one small worn leather bag, the same bag he arrived with by boat 45 years earlier. I knew that he had entered pure ecstasy but Heaven's gain impoverished the human race more than they could ever measure, for men such as this do not come often among us. I was silent a long time in his loss and denied my grief. Greatness had passed from us unnoticed, and yet the heavens roared in a single voice in one almighty hymn of wonder that moment when this simple man came barefoot before the throne of God. If there lies within us true goodness then Paul was the incarnation of it. A child with such unbridled delight, limitless. Everyone who met Paul just wanted to know him more. He was a magnet for everything that lived. Animals, birds, children and adults, he saw into them all. When you were with him, the whole of him was present to you in the most healing way. And in this man dwelt a holiness I had not seen before since Albert the Trappist.

In 1997, after caring for hundreds of young people dying of AIDS, Ronan and I watched one of our own die a most devastating and unspeakable death. Nothing would be served by describing the nine month journey of Sammy Ndwaru. I had known him since he was four years old. Now at 21, his unusual beauty had been ravaged and the husk of his living corpse struggled to breathe. We fed him with a straw, a drop at a time. Fr Tom Hogan, a veteran in Africa, spent time with him holding his wasted hand and talking with him in his own language. Lejiren was on one of his visits and he washed Sammy, cleaned him, and stayed with him every night through the pain and fear. He called him by his Kikuyu name Njoro, and Lejiren took much of the fear away. Once, when a nurse was trying to put in an intravenous drip, Sammy started to cry and Lejiren kissed his forehead and smiled and spoke to him in broken Kikuyu, making him laugh. Every time Sammy's daughter would come, Lejiren would sit Sammy up, put a hat on his head to hide the sores on the dull grey scalp, and make sure he was okay. He was very frail so Lejiren sat with him, propping him up.

Ronan too spent time alone in Sammy's last difficult journey. One night shortly before I had to leave for Europe, Sammy said to me he did not want to be here without me and he wanted to go home. I knew what he meant and said a quiet prayer to Paul asking him to hold Sammy in his arms.

Later that night Sammy gave his last breath and I lifted his 40 kilogram body into my arms and the pain had left his face. I kissed him goodnight and fell on my knees by his bed. In that moment everything I was seemed to leave my body and the weight of it all just passed through me. The futility of such violent suffering and loss, the utter shit of it all, filled me at once, and in a tidal wave of loss I fell into the tempest of helplessness. I felt utterly useless, desolate. There were emotions in me that have no words for them, no description of the darkness that came over me and the sense of futile barren hopelessness.

There within the loss of so much joy the faith within me was washed away in a despair that I had not prepared for or conceived. I held this withered hand, now cold, and in me raged a grief, a loss that threw me beneath the sewers of hell into a cold pit of numb rejection, disbelief and rage. I was too bereft to feel anger or revulsion. I was disgusted and unable to breathe. Throughout what seemed like hours of despair I knelt by Sammy's bed crying through gasps of breath, my sensations passing into memory and trembling. In my desolation there was in my eyes only blackness, but not the blackness when your eyes are shut, just a nothingness. I remember choking and trying to breathe but I couldn't. It was the middle of the night and I had already bent Sammy's hand, but I could not manage to draw breath. It was only after a few minutes that I felt Sarune's crippled fingers on the back of my neck.

He was very slowly speaking to the invisible. He was talking in an old dialect of Maasai and his words were soft and calm and belonged to the other world. He was like an electrical current and his touch began to draw my shattered, smashed being to itself. There was from within him something that came within me and I have no words to explain or describe the destruction of darkness. It was simply as if the abyss I had fallen into was very quietly filled with light. It was an effortless thing, just as all love is effortless. In the hours that passed Sarune was simply there, stiller than silence, more present than my own pulse. He was simply there. He held my hand and in him flowed the One, whatever the One is. Sarune was of the Engidon, the mystical seers of the old Maasai. Their ways are almost lost and few see them any more but in him flows the primeval energy ways long lost to us. Nowhere can man find a quieter or more untroubled retreat than in his own soul and Sarune lived within his own soul.

I have seen Sarune do many things I have no explanation for. We seem to like explanations, but I have learnt that they do not carry us very far. Everything that matters is not really about that. Sammy's daughter died of AIDS a few months later.

The many Japanese volunteers who worked with ICROSS in Africa were Buddhists. They understood the mysticism that pervaded the old tribes. Japanese culture was as old as theirs. They immediately related to the tranquillity and harmony of rural Africa. Unlike Western volunteers they related to the very different understanding of time and space. There was no need to achieve, compulsion to analyse, no thinking in straight lines. The Japanese had a profound respect for the ancient tribes and a healthy distance from many of the process management models being imported by the development industry.

By 1996 ICROSS programmes in Kenya had four long term donors. The Japanese Government was supporting a wide range of holistic projects from our surgical team and women's groups. A small group in the UK called The Little Way had supported our work among malnourished children since 1983. The Little Way was one of the only groups that understood the need for long term relationships with micro programmes often run by very old missionaries and doctors across the poor world. The third was Comic Relief, who were a young, cutting edge response to poverty. Will Day was a dynamic, passionate expert on Africa with a lot of experience, not least in Karamoja Desert where we both cut our teeth starting out. Will had been in a horrific car accident, breaking bones in 12 places, and he almost died. It did not help that he was six foot five inches tall.

The fourth long term support to our programmes was ICROSS in Ireland. Rebecca Burrell was a gentle and kind girl who came to see Dr Joe and I while I was on a trip to Dublin in 1990. She wanted to see how she could help. In time, she turned our tiny group into a real fundraising programme. She gradually took over from Dr Joe as the head of ICROSS in Ireland, while he remained the guiding light and energy of all we had.

A small group of close friends moved mountains. My childhood friend from Terenure, Kevin Niall, followed up corporate grants which were vital in our efforts to prevent infectious disease. He also followed applications to the Irish Government that had funded many primary health programmes.

Rebecca was unstoppable and her energy was infectious. Her best friend Jean came with her on one of many trips to Africa. As usual I stayed out of the way and let Africa speak for itself. Rebecca and Jean met the Maasai mothers and children and just as I had been they became enchanted and fell in love with the magic of the people and the primeval joy that fills them. These donors all had something in common. They were involved at a deeper level than themselves. They were engaged because of something more profound than wanting to do good. Ronan, Paul, Lemoite, Sarune, those close to me all had something in common too—they related at a deeper level.

Every night I meditated for a few hours after the Maasai had gone asleep. I was able to reach an awareness that would close down my senses and place myself in a state of deep stillness, lowering my heart beat. This had been a practice I learnt from Albert in the Cistercian Trappist monastery many years before.

The more you practise inward stillness the more you become a path for internal energy. In a sense this is autotelic—the energy is self-generating and internally evolving. There is a great difference between states of calmness and internal levels of mystical meditation. It has nothing to do with religion and everything to do with who we are. It is the portal that connects us to inner light. My inner life was the centre of my world and the harmony of everything else lay in its union with that inner state. It was an awareness and a disposition.

In Buddhism the pursuit of a life of compassion is the middle path to enlightenment. In Eastern mysticism seeing beyond the static of our preoccupations and letting go opens the way for inner joy. Every tradition converges, unites in a single undiluted truth. It is the followers and priests that institutionalise simple truths and wage war over their certitude. There is nothing more dangerous than religious certitude, no matter how it is masked in the name of God, freedom, or fighting terrorism.

The naked truth lies in the way of love and the way of compassion. This transcends religions.

***

My contemplative life continued to grow and was enriched by the energies around me, close friends, a daily life full of dynamic challenges and surprises, laughter and a deep vein of human suffering. There was music and art, creativity and passion. I loved languages and our research was demanding and intellectually rewarding. We are power and every day I was seeing new ways of discovering that power and channelling it. Of course there were failures and disappointments as well, but for the most part I was loving every second.

In the winter of 1999 I went to Chartres in France, a favourite haunt of mine, and one of those places so full of interior light that I go there as often as possible. There are places in this world that are deeply infused with presence, and the ancient glade of the druids was at Chartres. In Roman times the mystical rites were celebrated there and by the 4th century there was a place of hermits and stillness. Chartres is shrouded in mystery and has been for me a place of raw delight. I have brought my closest friends there and held their hands as they sat in awe. The canopy of the firmament domed across the vast expanse of an African night, the sacred and majestic are all about us.

On this particular evening I was listening to vespers at the back of the great cancelled eve. It was dark and raining outside but the music and the majesty were awe inspiring. As I was drifting somewhere between the voices and the sensations of the moment I heard a voice.

'Excuse me, sorry to bother you, could you please take my picture?' I raised my head and smiled.

'Of course,' I replied. 'Where would you like me to take it?' I asked, as I accepted his camera.

'I don't know, wherever.'

I offered him a few suggestions and told him that he was in one of the greatest gothic structures of all and that this was no ordinary place. I showed him the three lancet interior windows of life in sapphire blue that survived the great fire in 1194. I showed him the crypt that goes back to the 8th century and the druid well. He became at first interested then curious, then by the time I told him about the tree of life he was enthralled. An hour had gone by and he invited me for a drink. It was raining and dark and it was not until we reached a small bistro that I first saw him clearly. We reintroduced ourselves.

He was Carlo Manuel Antonio Cavelli Zacadelli. He was Italian and looked like a Caravaggio. Carlo was to become a very close friend in the following months as we explored Northern Italy and the alpine slopes. He snowboarded and I skied. Carlo had a wickedly dark sense of humour, an insatiable appetite for extreme sports, and a creative streak expressed in his amazing photography.

He had an encyclopaedic knowledge of the European masters and a taste for Greek mythology and sculpture. He opened my eyes to another world and his wild vivacious side brought us often to the edge of cliffs, literally, as he triple-spinned with the agility of a cat to the next cliff face. Carlo laughed from deep within his stomach and his attempts to teach me snowboarding met with the same success as my teaching him to avoid aggressive hockey-stops on hard snow. Because a thing seems difficult for us we should never assume that it cannot be done by someone else. This was the case with mid-air reverse spins on a thin board. Carlo rarely did things slowly and he had Italian emotional drivers that permeated through expressions, smiles and dancing.

There were interests we did not share. He was interested in fashion and trends, I was interested in French theatre. He liked a lot of modern music, my tastes were more ethnic and classical, so we learnt from each other. I listened to more Spanish guitar and jazz, and he listened to my Buddha bar compilations and tribal music. Carlo did everything well, not least talk. He could talk the his way through a stone wall and even when he had annoyed someone his smile always ended up melting them anyway. Carlo and I delighted in meeting each other's friends and it was only a matter of time before he started visiting Africa and he fell in love with it. Like most of my friends Carlo was an adventurer, a natural explorer, full of questions, and he had an artistic streak that touched every fibre of his being.

He awoke within me new horizons and opportunities and taught me to see through different eyes. His gentleness and tenderness created an affection and delight in me which gave birth to a very different me—one I had never known before. His sensuality and energy was always enthralling and mysterious, wild and passionate, and I was delighted that he had made me realise I was still learning about myself and who I was.

On one occasion we had a falling out and like most personal conflicts neither of us remembers why. For over two years we did not meet and then by chance

I was in London late one night in a bar. Carlo put his arms around me and smiled, and it was as if we had never argued. The friendship awoke within me so much delight and fun, it was always marvellous, magical, and as inspiring as Chartres.

CHAPTER NINE

'If you want others to be happy, practise compassion. If you want to be happy, practise compassion. There is no need for temples, no need for complicated philosophies. My brain and my heart are my temples; my philosophy is kindness.'
- *The Dalai Lama*

By late 1999, ICROSS had expanded its work into three more districts in Kenya. I was advising international health programmes, travelling in South East Asia, and sharing the ideas that we had demonstrated in Africa. While there, I had more opportunities to learn about Vedic and Eastern thought. Buddhist philosophy related closely to the oral traditions of the old tribes in East Africa and I felt increasingly comfortable in India and Thailand. I was within easy reach of the Indian sub-continent from East Africa and for a decade was to develop close ties with colleagues and friends across India. There were many differences between India and Africa though, not least the fact that I felt safer. Walking through Bombay at night was a pleasure, whereas I would never risk walking through any African city in the moonlight.

ICROSS developed policies and strategies to reflect the distinct differences between our ideas and other approaches to international aid. We found that we had a lot in common with many of our partner organisations. We were part of a dozen alliances and networks lobbying for change, and our partnerships led to increased political awareness.

ActionAid, *Médecins Sans Frontières*, Save the Children and others were challenging broader issues and the causes of poverty. There were growing reasons why we had to become more engaged. The figures were compelling. There are two worlds that are diverging exponentially; the rich world and a world increasingly reaching new extremes of unimaginable poverty, and there were some uncomfortable but unavoidable truths.

We all recognised that something needed to be done to not only highlight and address these problems, but to work towards solving them. The facts were boggling. The richest 50 million people in Europe and North America had the same income as 2.7 billion poor people. The slice of the cake taken by 1% was the same size as that handed to the poorest 57%. The world's 497 billionaires in 2001 registered a combined wealth of $1.54 trillion, well over the combined gross national products of all the nations of Sub-Saharan Africa ($929.3 billion) or those of the oil rich regions of the Middle East and North Africa ($1.34 trillion). It was also greater than the combined incomes of the poorest half of humanity.

12% of the world's population was using 85% of its water, and they all lived in the rich world. 10.6 million people died in 2003 before they reached the age of five. This is the same number as the child population in France, Germany, Greece and Italy. The total wealth of the top 8.3 million people around the world rose 8.2% to $30.8 trillion in 2004, giving them control of nearly a quarter of the world's financial assets. In other words, about 0.13% of the world's population controlled 25% of the world's assets in 2004, and the gap between the rich and the poor was growing every day.

Starvation is a terrible indicator of extreme poverty. If efforts are only directed at providing relief or aid, or improving food production or distribution, then the structural root causes that cause hunger, that create poverty and dependency, would continue. The political and economic determinants that cause the cycles of poverty remain the primary drivers of the engines that drive the poor into deeper traps of disease, misery and suffering, economic decline and separation from the rich world.

ICROSS had not been proactive on the international stage other than with our medical research. It would never be enough to simply establish effective and concrete methods of meaningful health care if the map itself was intrinsically wrong. Unless we were able to also place our limited efforts in context, our holistic strategy would have one eye closed—closed to the reality of why these diseases were emerging and why those we worked with were being plunged into a deeper, more insidious, yet avoidable future.

The spirals were slowed but the trends continued to decline, despite repeated rhetoric, and while the United States increased aid budgets, the overheads remained absurd and the agendas were openly strategic and neo-colonial. The Irish, Canadians and Scandinavians were historically good at listening to other cultures, but others were less gracious and assumed a knowledge they did not possess. The danger with importing template solutions was the inevitable failure that followed.

***

In one late night discussion I was talking with friends in the Foreign Office in London. One of them chided me that I was criticising political apathy, but what did I know of the agendas and manifestos of the politicians I was criticising? I confessed that I was ignorant of their stance or their strategies.

By the following week I had joined all the major parties in the UK and the Labour Party in Ireland, and started collecting various International Development Policies from friends in Paris, Munich, Washington and Tokyo. I spent a lot of time trying to understand the European and American development policies, talking to those who were inside the system. By mid-2000 I had begun to feel that ICROSS should become increasingly involved in influencing donor policies and international strategies. Any integrated approach to fighting poverty should, by definition, engage in all social change. We underlined our mission statement, which was to reduce disease, suffering and poverty among the poorest people on earth. Our projects were to be implemented through the values and beliefs of the people themselves. Together we would create self-reliance and work towards long term positive change.

Positive change, however, needs us to challenge ideas that do not promote equality and models that do not create an equal world. International aid was steeped in a racism and prejudice that operated from a stereotype of all things African. I was experiencing more and more that all too often the imbalance and games of power meant that discussions with poor nations were mere exercises, in diplomacy and futility.

The Irish Minister for International Development was Liz O'Donnell, who was uncompromising in her fight to increase Ireland's international contribution. Liz became a friend and advisor over the years, as did Lord Nick Rea, a medical doctor with experience in Africa and London's inner city. ICROSS was now becoming much more than just an organisation working in Africa. ICROSS was becoming a concept, an idea. The approach was a set of values, which was shared and advocated by a large and evolving international community. The values were not new but they were based on the belief that we were all born to be happy, all born as miracles, and within us was the power to change our destiny. Nelson Mandela, Desmond Tutu and Bono were among those challenging the attitude and hypocrisy of the Lords of Poverty. Many international organisations campaigned across a range of issues, while at the same time most of their budgets came from the very governments they were criticising.

The rich were not listening to the poor and all too often donors dictated and decreed rather than shared. Vulnerable African countries were often at the mercy of draconian structural readjustment programmes and expensive loans. For every $1 in aid, they were paying back $3 in interest-servicing loans. Small organisations across the world were trying their best to make an impact but the fabric of Africa was being torn apart by unfair trade and exploitation of countries that had no bargaining power. The core of our approach was to listen and work from and through tribal and community beliefs. The solutions would not be ours, they would belong to the philosophies and world views of the people. In other words, the approach would not be controlled by outsiders or those who had the money, but by the people themselves. Power and control would be African or local, not driven by agendas determined in a country the people had never seen. This proved an unpopular idea with donors who wanted policies and strategies influenced by their own, often well meaning, politics.

Most international aid budgets operate between two and five year cycles. The vast majority of grants are for two or three years. At the end of this there are expectations of sustainable health programmes. The absurdity of a criterion establishing sustainable strategies in desert areas with no cash economy escaped many bureaucrats. The irony that no country in the Western world had any sustainable health system was lost on people with little freedom to follow reason. Many of the policies that underpinned international development had no foundation in evidence or common sense. Many of the short lived funding initiatives existed as the result of political planning and lobbying, the evidence pointing to what were real priorities was irrelevant. ICROSS and many small organisations struggled with funding priorities that had no connection with the evidence of people's needs. If change was going to happen it would need realistic, long term commitment, and it would require international partnerships that rose above party politics or donor interests.

Desmond Tutu had started to challenge the hypocrisy of the West spending more on chocolate than on eradicating poverty, and the United States, whose military budget was many times what was needed to end world hunger. In my own lectures I became increasingly proactive in encouraging students and colleagues to become personally active themselves.

I argued that there are many levels of political action. I have never been drawn to protests or campaigns. Bringing justice into the world requires our action, not necessarily our complaining. We can be involved in Amnesty, but what are we going to do to heal the tortured, protect the weak, fight against cruelty? I increasingly believed that we needed to be more closely involved in fighting the oppression of the poor. That meant finding out more about what was going on. We need to have integration, giving us balance that also means awareness; information needed to become knowledge through wisdom, a wisdom that calls us to informed action. ICROSS began reaching out to commercial sex workers who were being exploited, providing help and support to old people, and legal aid and advice to people who were dying of AIDS. It meant creating a rights based approach to an increasingly dynamic response to people's problems. The connecting thread between all of these issues we had been addressing was the right of every human being to be happy.

We moved away from the narrow ideas of health care and began to think that human rights were a vital part of health and happiness.

In the pursuit of happiness the Dalai Lama said, 'If you want others to be happy, practise compassion. If you want to be happy, practise compassion. There is no need for temples, no need for complicated philosophies. My brain and my heart are my temples; my philosophy is kindness.' This was a wisdom the Dalai Lama has continued to share, a vision of personal joy and living compassion. Our true natures are to be happy, and there is not enough joy in the world. The happiness of our lives depends upon the quality of our thoughts, so it is up to us to enrich them.

At the same time we began advocacy programmes in 2000, ICROSS also began talking in schools. While many of us had shared our research at conferences and in international journals, we felt the time had come to explore new ways of sharing and lobbying. We created a series of web sites in Canada and England, Ireland and Africa. New partners like Aid Link and ActionAid in Ireland shared many of our concerns and together with the Elton John Foundation we extended support to the terminally ill and to AIDS orphans and other children made vulnerable by the ravages of famine and poverty. A growing network of people were beginning to do the same thing and Billy Willbond in Canada was already sending millions of dollars of emergency medical equipment and wheelchairs to South America, Angola, Malawi, Afghanistan and Uganda. At the same time I had handed over the management of our programmes to African teams who could do so much more than I ever would in creating new opportunities and possibilities.

We were seeing extraordinary progress and dynamic shifts in the patterns of disease. Our work was making a difference and more interest in our methods drew new support. Despite the odds, a lot of our long term work was demonstrating compelling evidence of real change. With renewed hope and growing curiosity, we extended our programmes to new tribes in the Interior. We took on new diseases and new challenges. We were increasingly amazed at the wisdom and knowledge that lay unexplored and unused within the great cultures of Africa.

CHAPTER TEN

'The secret is to see everything you do as wonder and everything you are as magic, because you are mystery.'
- *Sarune*

In Africa, life is full of surprises. One hot summer's day, a few Japanese volunteers were being visited by an official from Tokyo. They went to visit one of our training projects deep in Maasai land. I had gone north into Sudan to see one of our child survival programmes, but when I came back I found that the training hadn't happened. Everyone had vanished into the bush. A young mother had fallen asleep under a tree and a large female baboon had snatched her sleeping baby. For three days the Maasai pursued the large troop of baboons, and when they finally tracked the female she surrendered the baby with little fuss. She had been fed and there was not a scratch on her.

On another occasion a visitor had rented a land rover and had gone with Lemoite to northern Samburu, near Lake Turkana. The enthusiastic visitor climbed out of the car to get a good photograph of a clutch of ostrich eggs, but got a little too close, and the female charged. The frightened photographer jumped back in the car, but before driving away, a kick tore a deep hole in the new Land Rover's passenger door. It is never wise to get between a mother and her young.

I started living in manyattas in the early 1980s, which is a small collection of tiny cow dung huts surrounded by a thorn fence to keep out wild animals. We would have the baby goats sleep under our bed (there was only one bed). There were no windows, no running water. Cooking was done on the earthen floor and we lived as people have done for thousands of years. It was here I found the happiest monastery of the heart and my cloister was the vast endless canopy of the African night; a billion stars, witness to the Creator and the symphony of a pulsing chant to the heaving of the abyss. The grandeur of the creation spoke to my heart, and the majesty of its perfection was more eloquent than any philosophy.

Ever since we had our first manyattas in Samburu, one of the young warriors who lived among us was Lejiren. Lejiren had many parts, many personalities. He was always different, and a little crazy. He had mood swings and he could be dangerous. Once he attacked four men who were trying to steal goats late one night. He had cut the ear off one and was fearlessly attacking the others when I intervened and let them go. Lejiren never had a capacity for fear—he simply wasn't afraid of anything. This often got him into trouble and he had been in jail several times. He never seemed to feel pain. Above all, however, everyone who knew him knew his childlike sense of delight in everything. Everything was a new pleasure, each day was a precious discovery, and he was thrilled with the smallest wonder. He was gentle with animals, kind to the old, but pure magic with children, any children. He had the power to entrance children and make them laugh, even children who were afraid and very sick. Lejiren possessed so many innate gifts, and if the cards he was dealt were different, he would have had a very successful career in anything he put his mind to.

Lejiren was pure Samburu and was unfettered by convention. Like the native Australian people, the Samburu often just go wandering on 'walkabout'. Sometimes you might see Lejiren, but then he would be gone for weeks, only to reappear suddenly, always unannounced. Once we had a guard at one of the remote clinics in Turkana who disappeared, but three years later he returned, wondering why he could not have his job back; the clinic had long been handed over to the community and the Ministry of Health. Lejiren, however, would appear and reappear over the years, sometimes to tell us he was going to jail, sometimes just looking after his small herd of goats.

I had more freedom to travel around now, consulting and lecturing, and whenever I was in Ireland I would spend as much time with Dr Joe as I could. Joe was now in his late eighties. He had seen ICROSS grow from a small, tentative project into a viable initiative that touched the imaginations of many. Like most of us, Joe was involved in many charities and organisations but his heart had a special place for ICROSS. He was incapable of frustrating or boring anyone and everyone he met wanted more. Joe commanded a love and respect I have not seen elsewhere. Joe always had a new book, a fascinating insight; he was always learning and questioning, always animated and engaged in everything. That connectedness with the great drama of life and fascination with everything was always exciting to behold. We all need renewal, all need acceptance and encouragement, and Joe gave it to me in abundance. My hero has always been this gentle, humble man with nothing to prove. His integrity and courage have always shone bright and even when he fell off his bike, ending up in hospital, he was asking everyone else how they were, reaching out, seeing beyond himself into everyone else's needs. After that accident though, Joe wisely stopped riding a bicycle. He got a tricycle instead!

By 2001 I had started sculpting life size bronzes, after a long break. There had been famines and droughts, epidemics and malaria, amoebic dysentery, and a lot of travel to Asia to take care of first. With the African teams now taking on most of the work, I had more time to write, research, study and work on the development of ICROSS internationally. There was a steady stream of friends like Ronan, who launched new programmes, dropping by, and Francesca and Carlo arrived, frequently unannounced, always knowing they were at home with me. I spent more time with friends and less time in the bush, realising that the time was right to let younger energies work with their own people. My stillness grew, as did my creativity, but there were new challenges and exciting new horizons to be explored. I tried to treat every act of my life as if it were my last. Everything that exists is, in a manner, the seed of that which will be, and in this knowledge I believed more than ever in the necessity to celebrate what we had.

Mum and Dad visited every couple of years and saved up to come and spend time in a place where they were celebrated in their old age. Africa loves the old and rejoices in them. Mum and Dad had a stream of visitors and the visits became longer over the years. One time when they arrived, Lejiren was on one of his visits and entertained everyone with jokes, and a sense of fun that warmed the coldest hearts. While he possessed many graces, Lejiren was also a compulsive thief and stole anything he could, whenever he could.

He was banished from the camp at the Ngong Hills, back to Samburu, after it was discovered he stole an envelope containing money from Mum's bedroom. We never found the missing $700, but as usual Lejiren had crossed a new line, only this one would be harder to return from. We often tend to think of people as good or bad, decent or useless. In real life we all have shades of darkness and shadows of light. We are contradictions and paradoxes. If we can't easily fathom a person's complexity, we step back and fade to grey. If we are confronted with inconsistencies or confusion we desert the situation. In Africa, I have found that people seem to be able to tolerate the failures, sins and uncertainties in each other because they do not think in black and white. There is a pervading understanding that we are all good and bad, gentle and harsh, and within the same piece of creation there can be great goodness and also things that are dark, yet which do not diminish the light.

In the Western world, we live in a culture of gossip and scandal where time and energy are spent in displaying the sins and frailties of each other instead of the beauty we can accomplish together. Our media thrives on blame and fear. We praise trivia and applaud mediocrity, pretending depth is too difficult for us. It is this vehicle of education that has created the image of Africa that has so coloured the Western mind. The average perception of Africa and Asia is so crippled by negative stereotypes that one of the emerging tasks for us all is to change the understanding and attitude towards others. Prejudice and intolerance is expressed in many ways; paternalism, arrogance, intellectual superiority, unspoken assumptions, and the language of 'they', the culture of blame, pre-grasped understanding, and presumption of knowledge, condescension, and pity. In many of these responses there is often good will and genuine intent to be of help. But there is often a tacit assumption that Africans are less honest and less able and it is an assumption that is often subtle and veiled in the language of partnership.

***

Every few years we stepped back and evaluated the direction of our programmes. More importantly, we questioned the model and the ideas that were behind an international community relieving starvation and suffering. We challenged our assumptions and the reasons we were involved in health care. While we were seeing changes in the patterns of disease, were we doing enough? While we were measuring demonstrable improvements in the lives of many people, we asked how we could be more effective. A continuous evaluation process of our epidemiological and preventive care programmes was important. The model we were evolving involved lessons and values that we thought would be of inherent value and applicable in all development programmes. Many of those involved in ICROSS were also working in other development organisations internationally. Many of the specialists, including myself, were regularly contracted to advise in the design, evaluation, implementation or monitoring of large scale programmes. We began to see that many of the lessons learnt in integrated holistic long term programmes might be applied elsewhere.

At the same time we needed to place our work in the context of international strategies, so we were diligent in integrating the World Health Organisation,

UNAIDS, UNICEF and other multilateral priorities and aims. In each country we also built in the national policies for public health and primary health care development. These processes formed the core of five year plans and strategic plans that helped prepare ICROSS to meet the new challenges being faced by rapidly changing conditions. The process of the 'Africanisation' of our main programmes was finally completed in 2001 with all the management and administration of field projects run by local teams. I was free to concentrate on disease research, the development of new programmes, and to explore other opportunities to share the ICROSS approach in other contexts. We were receiving hundreds of requests for advice every year, so Ronan and I spent an increasing amount of time sharing our methodology.

The core elements remained disarmingly simple, though not as easy to implement as it would appear. There were people driven agendas that often did not meet the priorities of donor guidelines. There was long term responsibility rather than short term funding. There was cultural control from the community, not adaptation to Western models, and there was scientific evidence led planning, not management process-driven projects. Evaluation was about the impact on real life, not how successfully processes were followed in implementation plans. The model stressed donor as well as local transparency. It relied on local, not foreign language decision processes, and planning as well as community belief systems rather than imported values and agendas.

There are many international guidelines governing the ethics of medical research. These range from the Nuremburg Code and Helsinki Declaration to the Convention on Human Rights and the ethical codes of the health professions. A growing number of those in international health believe we need standards of practice that would govern the way in which international aid is given. At present there are no international standards that control or govern the quality, standard or practice of working among vulnerable populations.

There are many excellent organisations that aspire to and attain the highest standards of health care and management. Many of these bodies like CARE, Médecins Sans Frontières, Oxfam, Concern, Merlin, ActionAid, and GOAL operate to standards of excellence that can be independently verified. There are however many examples of amateur, poorly conceived, misguided and dangerous projects that exist simply because an organisation has money. It is important that we introduce, within the international framework of global aid, minimum standards and a register of best practice. This is part of the strategic direction of ICROSS that has been developed by our partners, colleagues and collaborators.

My own role in this process began in 1983 with initial discussions with Professor David Morley, Professor John Waterlow, Dr David Nabarro of the London School of Hygiene and Tropical Medicine, and Dr Ian Monroe of *The Lancet*. Dr Tom O'Riordan and I floated the early idea of an interdisciplinary forum that would work to evolve new criteria and standards that would not only enforce best practice but be able to score international agencies and health programmes' performance, cost effectiveness, cost to benefit ratio, and long term impact. In the early 1980s, the culture of evidence led decision taking was eclipsed by political positioning.

Now, the global shift towards transparency and accountability influenced by both the Clinton Report on Africa in 2002 and the British White Paper on Poverty in 2004 created a new opportunity to develop more effective ways of working together towards lasting shifts in eradicating poverty. Exciting new avenues are currently being developed by a series of global movements. While ICROSS is part of movements like 'Make Poverty History', the networks of groups advocating policy changes and international alliances, real change will come from the think-tanks, advisory groups and consultancy structures that influence the security and financial decisions made at cabinet level. It is only when we begin reconstructing the way political advisors understand and present issues of poverty that actual paradigm shifts will take place.

After a lot of study and an immense amount of research and thought, Ronan Conroy and I finally came up with a framework for best practice. All international aid must, in my view, meet seven minimum requirements to be valid and ethical. These criteria were developed over time and are part of a forthcoming series of works on rethinking the international development model:

1. Independent reviews of the transparency, accountability, governance and value of programmes are essential. This includes the assessment of the knowledge, design, plan, community understanding and ethical integrity of policies and interventions.

2. There must be informed consent and respect for the autonomy and rights of recipients of all aid as equal voices in all processes concerning them. Informed sharing of all procedures, ideas, choices,

and alternatives in every situation especially disasters, famines, and emergencies is vital.

3. The aid must be of demonstrable and requested social benefit and value to the communities as they define value themselves. This must be externally verifiable.

4. All development has to exist within the local cultural, religious, ethnic and social values. It should be within the epistemology, belief systems, language context, and social construct, as expressed and interpreted by the people themselves.

5. All programming and policy must be explained by evidence and scientifically validated fact, not political or institutional opinion.

6. Target communities and groups should be involved in every decision at every level and should be involved as equals in the financial, administrative and planning processes.

7. There must be a respect for local realities, choices, selection of teams, sharing of power and openness of information.

CHAPTER ELEVEN

'We may have found a cure for most evils; but we have found no remedy for the worst of them all—the apathy of human beings.'
- *Helen Keller*

Over the years I had tried to understand something of the poverty in Europe by attempting, if only for a moment, to experience living on the streets. This was never a very good way to learn because it was only for a few nights and I could never understand the long term degradation and erosion of self and personal worth, but I did learn some things and was given some fresh perspectives and ideas. I first attempted this experience in the late 1980s and have done it several times since, in both London and Paris.

I had been on a lot of spiritual retreats and practised meditation, and as a result had learned to welcome and experience surreal spiritual experiences that lifted me out of everyday existence and opened up new horizons on a more astral plain. But I am from Europe, and grew up in an affluent environment, so I knew that in order to get in touch with the essence of existence, of joy and suffering, I had to experience life in all its forms, for myself, to gain a spirituality formed from living without possessions. I knew that if spirituality needed to be fed from monasteries, it was not real for me. I could gain spirituality, but I would never really know how people in less well off circumstances, who lived a much tougher, more painful existence, felt.

I needed to find out what it was like to be as invisible as the people the world constantly ignored, to understand how they felt, so that I could help them more. I have experienced, in one way or another, a lot of sensory deprivation over the years. I have been blinded, and incapacitated through disease, and have found myself caught in severe famines suffering from malnutrition. I know what it is like to be terribly anorexic from famine, having once gone down to six and a half stone in weight from 11 and a half, and to feel a total sense of worthlessness as a result. This is not recommended, but it was the situation we were in at the time. But I also know that as a person I rarely have any negative feelings and am almost always happy. I wanted to empathise and understand a lot more. Rather than an intellectual understanding of how people suffer, I wanted a deeper feeling of what it is like to seem so worthless. I wanted to try to understand human suffering more, because better treatment comes from better understanding. This is why we prefer to live with the villagers and tribes in Africa, rather than in a separate, more comfortable place. We live with the people, eat what they eat, drink what they drink, and suffer what they suffer, so that we can better understand what they go through, and can offer better, practical, experience based treatment as a result.

I would often find myself in ornate and prestigious buildings, giving lectures to well to do and well off audiences, wearing top designer clothes, before heading to fancy restaurants to dine and talk to important, high profile people. But I would notice the other people walking by—the homeless, the poor, victims of the sex trade—and these people understood what it was like to not be seen, to be invisible and ignored by society, in much the same way as those suffering in Africa were unseen, unrecognised, ignored.

The idea started to form in my head. I have always been interested in how different people see things. From the Maasai mothers, to artists and poets, everybody has a unique view of the world, and I realised that I needed to see things as others saw them. I needed to see the world through the eyes of the poor and invisible. I decided to start an experiment, to see what it was like to be an outsider in society with nothing to call my own, and so I started to sleep rough on the streets, firstly in London, and then later in Paris.

I once gave a lecture to a prestigious crowd in London before heading back to my hotel, which was paid for by somebody else, and decided to leave everything and head out onto the streets with nothing but the clothes I was wearing. It was more for my own humility than anything else, because I felt I was just getting too far away from the reality of the people I was trying to help. I spent two nights sleeping rough before returning to my own life, and was to do the same thing many times in an attempt to feel what those who truly had nothing felt.

The majority of people I met living rough in London shifted in central London from being older wine drinking groups in the mid-1980s to being teenagers running away from home a decade later. I would generally sleep near Victoria train station because there was safety in numbers. There were areas where the rent boys would be and other places where the poorer ones would sleep, and there were areas where the long term groups had staked out. In the 1980s few had a pet dog to guard them but by the 1990s many did, and these dogs were well trained to protect their owners from being attacked, robbed or urinated on. I had stayed with the young drifters who were generally disorganised, and they generally travelled in couples. Many of them were just a little lost and had family problems, and most found their way back out of the begging spiral. A lot did drugs but most didn't.

It was here I had my first encounters with ladies of the night. They never walked alone, and rarely looked as tacky as on TV. Seline looked about 20 and was working the clubs. She asked me if I was alright. I looked cold and uncomfortable sitting on a step near the deserted bus stops. She offered me a cigarette, but I didn't smoke, so she told me there was a mobile soup kitchen over the other side of the station. She told me not to sit alone and to go and look for the people not carrying bottles. She walked me to a corner and pointed me in the right direction.

Every encounter and conversation I had with such girls over the years was like this. They were always caring, always concerned, rarely drunk. They were not like any of the stereotypes or portrayals I assumed. The first time I slept out on the streets one girl had bought me chips. Another time I was given a pen knife to protect myself.

I found out what it was like to sleep on cardboard boxes with filthy blankets with nothing to protect me from the weather or violent attacks. I was surrounded by drug addicts, crime, and all sorts of vice, and realised just how dangerous it was to be trapped in this lifestyle. Violence threatened around every corner, and if something happened, there would be nobody to miss you.

I wandered around the streets of London for days at a time, scavenging whatever I could, but barely eating, never washing, sleeping in dank and dark alleyways or on benches in parks or at bus stations, struggling to survive. Apart from the fear, which is constant, I began to feel a horrible, dull ache in my stomach. It was the feeling of being constantly hungry. Even if I had just managed to find something to eat, I would still feel this terrible hunger, because it just wasn't enough to make up for days with nothing at all to sustain me. This was real hunger, something I saw all too often in famines.

A lack of food brings about a change in your dietary patterns. If you don't get enough to eat, you don't move your bowels, and your stomach basically stops working. Your body becomes weaker and you actually start to look and act less than human. Forced to scavenge for scraps of food, you feel even less human. You become inferior, sub-human, and this brings about drastic changes that add to the effect. Your head begins to bow, making you look almost like you are grovelling before superiors, and you start to feel like you are being eroded, adding to your sense of unworthiness and meaninglessness. This inevitably becomes how people walking by see you. You are cold, damp and smelly, and you feel like shit all of the time. And people just can't see past your appearance or their preconceptions about you to see that beneath it all you are a human just like them; a human suffering and in need of help.

As I walked the streets in dirty, stinking clothes, with nowhere to go and nothing to hope for, what immediately hit me was the invisibility I had instantly incurred. It was instantaneous. Friends I had seen only days before were walking by without recognising me because like everybody else, they were averting their eyes. The moment the homeless person comes into our line of vision, our mind tells us to turn away, to not make eye contact, to ignore that person's very existence. As I sat on roadsides and stood in slums, it was as if I was wearing a mask all of a sudden. I was like the lower castes of India; I was actually not there, as far as ordinary people were concerned. I was, to them, sub-human.

I was shocked by this, but knew that I was really only scratching the surface of what it was like to be such a person, an invisible being that society would rather ignore. It was only an experiment for me, so I knew I could never fully understand. I was sleeping in dives in Hackney and Brixton, sharing space with the true homeless, meeting prostitutes and rent boys and the true down and outs. It was dangerous and dirty, and filled with a constant sense of fear, but I knew that it just wasn't real; that at any time I could return to my friends and enjoy the affluent surroundings of Chelsea and Knightsbridge if I really wanted. These other poor, dejected souls didn't have that choice. They were here for good. I was in learning mode, taking it all in, but these people go into a state of denial, a sort of comatose state whereby they don't feel like they have been rejected by society and by their fellow man because they come to think of this ragged, hungry person as someone else, not them. But in the long run, their self-worth is eroded until they become nothing but an empty forgotten shell of what was once a human being.

I experienced the same awful feelings on the streets of Paris where again I suddenly became invisible to everybody walking by, as if they refused to recognise my existence. Again I knew I could only experience so much. I knew I could stop kneeling on the streets begging, as is the tradition, and return to friends at the cafes along the Seine. But I did at least gain a new perspective. Even if it was only for short periods at a time, I began to understand how these people felt, and it wasn't good.

The impression left on my outlook was strong. I could not get over how, when I was on the streets, sleeping rough, I simply was not seen. Nobody wants to look at you, to see you as another human being. But what is worse is that after a while, you begin to do the same thing, to develop a cocoon to say, 'This is not me', making you invisible even to yourself. Having met a lot of prostitutes and rent boys in my time on the streets of both London and Paris, and having met many others over the years, some of whom have become good friends, what strikes me about them is that they readily place themselves outside of their own identities, refusing to acknowledge that it is them doing what they are doing, because it is the only way they know to deal with the awful lives they have to lead in order to survive.

This to me is a tragedy. No person should ever become invisible to another. I began to realise that we need to see every single person as somebody just as important as every other person; that we have to stop ignoring the rights and the suffering of others, because they are people just like us. Whether I was in Africa treating children with malnutrition or some awful disease, or sleeping rough on the streets of London, sharing a pile of cardboard boxes with tramps, or giving a lecture to a room full of academics in Dublin, I wanted to treat everybody as equal, no matter what they did, who they were, or where they were from.

Everybody needs the sympathy and empathy of others.

We need to see people as individuals, not as representatives of a group, or type. Sometimes it can be hard to see others as people, but try imagining that difficult person you know, for example, playing with their children, and you will see them in a different light. I try to keep the same view in everything I do. When I give a lecture, I imagine I am talking to an individual, and not to a room full of people. It is something we all need to do; to see that each person is an individual, a real person who feels the same things you do.

If there are no opportunities we can create them; if there are no doors open to us we can build our own doors, but this is only possible if we have enough self-worth and enough love in our lives to take the first step. We all need help and everything we do is linked profoundly with the friendship and encouragement we have in our lives.

My encounters with prostitutes while I was sleeping rough on the streets reinforced in me the need to show the world that every single person needs the sympathy we would like ourselves, because they are just people like us in the end. This is true the world over.

One of the most misunderstood groups in the AIDS epidemic in Africa was prostitutes. The politically correct mood of the moment renamed prostitutes with the more sanitised name of 'commercial sex workers', just as AIDS victims and patients would be called clients and lepers would be called persons with leprosy.

***

There are some people who walk through life who are self-empowered. These are people who invariably use positive language, are focused on others, are creators and healers. They are self-energising and self-realising. Usually such people achieve and build emotionally and dynamically. Autotelic personalities are people who rely internally for motivation, affirmation, acceptance and inspiration. They are relatively rare but they do exist. One such autotelic is Colin Meagle, a close friend I met originally through Rebecca. We instantly connected. The first thing you realise when meeting autotelic people is their positive energy, engagement with everyone, internal calm and a natural motherboard of intelligences operating in balance. In the study of happiness, autotelic people invariably are found to be innately, profoundly delighted most of the time. They are able to manage life's crises and problems so creatively and positively that even in tragedy they emerge enriched and reclaimed faster than others.

The nature of an autotelic is to construct reality and situations through positive inter-relationships, thus maximising experience all the time. They solve problems quickly because they focus on solutions, not the distractions that made the problem. They navigate routes to stress free living and do not get trapped by thought patterns that don't go forward. Colin is a perfect example. Like all of us, he has to cope with deadlines, let-downs and high pressure situations. He has to deal with bills and loud people, deceptions and hassles. Life has these things. Autotelic response, however, refuses to allow negative dynamics to become part of the interior life. Colin does not allow an insult or someone's anger into his head. The fact that he is a musician helps; there are many autotelics who have a musical intelligence.

He has a strong self-discipline and is an advanced practitioner in Aikido, with a real physical and spatial intelligence and personal calm. This too is typical in autotelics (the calmness, not the Aikido). Colin rarely talks about himself and his achievements, whereas people who need external affirmation need to talk about themselves and find approval and affirmation externally.

***

ICROSS was working on new ways to reduce harm and infection due to female circumcision. Working with traditional tribes, one requires above all respect and patience in sharing potential ideas and suggestions. Not all innovation was as easy as reducing neonatal tetanus. Body scarification and circumcision had roots deep within personal identity and self-image.

As we were developing female circumcision programmes and expanding safe motherhood we began to see long term results from immunising infants over decades.

Meanwhile in 2002, I received an unexpected e-mail inviting me to a Terenure College reunion. I could not believe it was 25 years since I had left school, as it only seemed like yesterday. Carlo was still trying to teach me snowboarding and Fabricio was still trying to get me to understand flamenco and wear bright colours. I was talking the same week on the new faces of poverty to a small group in Paris so I was at least going to be in Europe, and managed to reach Dublin. It was strange to recognise the boys in the masks of men and the kindnesses of time and lifestyle within their countenance. It had been longer than I thought, and I felt like an alien dislocated from the world I had left behind. It was delightful to see that so many had done so very well, and it was a profound reminder of the brief moment we are in and the pleasure every day has been. I had remained close to many of my school friends who had worked together at creating the many successes we had together in Africa and Asia. Many were in my heart, and Tom, above all, shared all of my life despite living in America.

On the night of that reunion I met not just men who had lived blessed and fabulous lives in many places, but husbands and fathers who spoke with love and grace. We shared stories and memories, jokes and recollections. Long forgotten deeds were remembered and hands touched that had not felt each other in a generation. Among them was Ed Kelly who as I remembered played rugby in school. Ed put his hand on my shoulder and told me as we left that he would try and help what we were doing in Africa. He was a straight talker not accustomed to bullshit, so I knew that I would hear from him again.

A few months later Ed had rounded up his friends and drew together a new thrust of support. Ed was like me in many ways, determined, as relentless as an avalanche, as persistent and inevitable as a glacier. He set out to move our Irish organisation forward and within a year he was working with Rebecca Burrell and Jean Lowes in repositioning ICROSS in Ireland. While the African organisation had become well-established it was relying on the voluntary efforts of a handful of friends. ICROSS needed to evolve if it was going to support projects reaching over 250,000 people in Africa. Ed worked with our group pushing forward changes that would place ICROSS on a more stable footing and create a solid base from which to build the support desperately needed. Without this leap, ICROSS could not expand in Europe. I admired Ed's passion and had growing respect for his affection and love poured upon a family that was his joy. I saw perhaps what I could have been and smiled often at his pleasure playing with his children. Ed's daughter once asked me why every time I went to Ireland I wore exactly the same clothes. I explained I never carried luggage and had one set of clothes in each country, though I am not sure she believed me. A few other guys I went to school with joined us in bringing in more support and by 2003, Ed had roped in another classmate, Conor O'Kelly.

Conor created a new opportunity for ICROSS in the NCB sponsorship of ICROSS primary health programmes. This single act dramatically altered the five year plan of ICROSS in Africa, guaranteeing the diarrhoea control, safe motherhood and infant mortality programmes in a single partnership. At the same time Ed drew in another lifelong friend who went to school in Blackrock, Shane O'Neill.

Shane and his wife Sheelagh would visit our AIDS programmes in Africa and soon afterwards set up ICROSS in the UK. Within four years Ed was instrumental in achieving what I had failed to do, establishing a viable base of support in the UK.

Over the years we had developed a network of friends around the world, many of whom shared our passions and concerns about the trends within global development. There were many people quietly working towards a better world, creating positive change. Clare Hanbury ran the Child to Child health promotion programmes based in London She was a tireless advocate for children's rights. Clare was pure magic and always sensed need in others. She was one of life's positive forces and did not know the meaning of failure. She was one of the close circle of friends who always shared her home. I was always welcome, always wanted. It is the Clares of this life that allow you to do impossible things.

Most of Clare's friends were also involved in breaking the boundaries. Nick Mellor had co-founded MERLIN, Kate Harrison had been in Uganda and was working with Healthlink Worldwide, changing the way health care was being done across the poor world. Kate had three things—a profound insight into Africa, a deep understanding of the complexity of poverty, and a burning fire inside her to make a real difference. She was always able to work within the structures of development while at the same time gently challenging the assumptions and ideas behind many flawed policies. Kate was working with the dynamic and innovative International HIV/AIDS Alliance and our paths crossed frequently in our work with AIDS orphans and with other vulnerable children. Kate would be the editor of a collaborative book on the most vulnerable children that we would write for distribution across Africa.

As ICROSS became more engaged in the care of the terminally ill, an increasing number of communities sought our help. By mid 2003, ICROSS was reaching over 12,000 victims and the number was rising by the month. We drew together all our contacts and partners and managed to raise the funds to start new home care programmes along Lake Victoria in the districts of Bondo and Siayia. With help from the Canadian and Australian Governments we started training those caring for the dying and creating ways that women's groups could help orphaned children in their villages.

The task was mammoth, far bigger than we could have imagined. For a period we received support from the US funded Family Health International. It was run by the most gentle and honourable of men, John McWilliam. John turned out to be an old India hand. He had been a US Peace Corps volunteer in West Africa. In everything John was gracious and caring. John had the unenviable job of dealing with the American bureaucrats, something he did effortlessly. The politics of aid was about power and power was about money, those who had the money attempted to exert often undue influence on poor countries. It was always a delicate balance. The British were invariably more respectful and courteous than the Americans while the Scandinavians always tried to be polite to everyone, often inadvertently offending them instead.

By 2004 ICROSS had 42 projects scattered across the vast tracts of Kenya and five projects in Tanzania as well as providing assistance to health interventions in Cambodia, Uganda and Ethiopia. We were receiving 300 requests for technical advice a week and all the management was now completely local.

All Will Be Well was released in May 2004. Like *All Shall Be Well*, it was an extended version of my articles reflecting on the experiences I had in Africa, sharing the delight and laughter, hope and wonder. It sold very well but more importantly it created a new wave of interest in our work in both the UK and Ireland. Jennifer Glasse reformatted the second edition and within a few months we had gone into a third edition. It shared a little of the spirit and passion of Africa as well as the constant victory of kindness over cruelty and light over darkness. A series of media articles raised awareness of the plight of children living in extreme poverty and the efforts of ICROSS to reach them. Our renewed advocacy campaigns in Ireland and England raised over £1 million though we were now being stretched in Africa with malaria outbreaks, the start of drought and increased diarrhoeal infections in many areas. Ed Kelly and his friends shared our work with their close friends. Its cost effectiveness, low overheads, and impact appealed to people.

I was in Europe giving a lecture when I met a young Danish student who asked if he could get some advice on working in Africa. Morten Skovdal was 24, calm, placid and engaging. He was highly intelligent, well informed and like so many Danes, self-effacing. I was with Keith, an Irish friend from Dublin. We were both impressed by Morten's passion. He had volunteered in China, he had been in United World College in Norway, also spoke German, had wide interests, loved dancing. He had a great degree from LSE and asked all the right questions. We stayed in touch and I arranged that Morten could work in one of our AIDS programmes in Africa.

Within a month, Morten had networked our computer system, streamlined the office, slept in the slums, visited the toughest projects, given away all his money and most of his clothes and was settled in. He dealt with setbacks with a quiet calm, his mild manner and soft voice could be mistaken for meekness, but there was Viking in his blood and he was loving every problem, crisis and challenge. The more I grew to know Morten, the more I realised how far he had come. He had lost his mother to cancer when he was 12 and in many ways he made his way in the world alone. He was self-starting and learnt with the speed of a child. He fell in love with the Maasai, spending weeks at a time in the bush. After a few months Sarune gave him a name, Tadju. Tadju became more and more engaged in the harder part of our work, often spending time with people who were very ill and dying, often playing with the children, always working with humility and respect—precious qualities.

Out of nowhere I received an award, the International Person of the Year Award in Ireland in 2003. I am still not sure why. It was a wonderful evening and I borrowed Tom's shoes and a waiter's tie. The only thing of mine was my underwear. Tom had flown in from America. When the presenter Mary Kennedy asked me what kept me going, I replied 'prayer'. I did believe that without placing all the human suffering and tragedy at the feet of God, one would have to try and carry the meaningless suffering and poverty in one's own heart. Without stillness and inner balance, everything in life could be a source of anxiety. In experiencing joy from within, everything is really amazing.

Gay Byrne, Ireland's most famous presenter, came up to me after the award ceremony, smiled and he told me that that is one thing not mentioned these days on TV . . . prayer. My close friend Crispin Lowe came over from London and was charmed with the Irish ways. Crispin had a slightly innocent view of the Irish. He said one of the wonderful things about Dublin was that if you stood on a street corner with a map you would have lots of lovely Irish people coming over and offering directions, pointing you in any given direction. Hmm, depends on which street corner I guess. Crispin had come and seen our projects in Kenya and had always offered me a place to stay in London.

Terenure College had a new lease of life and was becoming yet again involved in our work. I was always very interested in getting young people passionate about Africa, because like their peers living in poverty, they were our tomorrow. Other friends and classmates had heard of our effort and became involved. Rebecca had drawn in more of her friends and there were little events across the country. At one function in Cork I met Eddie Hobbs, whose straight talking and honest analysis had awoken a nation in his series, 'Rip Off Ireland'. Eddie was a great help and had a big heart. David Weakliam continued to quietly inspire me and understood the challenges in a modern age. We shared our concerns and decided that one expression of hope might be to share the delight and wonder of Therese of Lisieux with a new generation. For her, union was a simple disposition of the heart, a cry of recognition and of love, embracing both trial and joy; it was a delight in everything. Faith for Therese was the strength by which a shattered world shall emerge into the light.

***

I started writing this book while on retreat with Colin in Glencolumbcille, West Donegal. It is so easy to create around such an autotelic open energy that only sees beauty, energy, grace, and light. The amount of positive energy created by some people is so strong that it eclipses that pettiness, drains and negatives instantly. It is only when we are energised by close friends that really see how extraordinary life is. We are transformed and renewed when we are with those we love; we are richer for being in their presence, we are flooded in the flow. In my life I am surrounded by the Toms, Joes and Ronans. I have Sarune and Elle my assistant, little Joe and Patrick. We are in so many ways changed by those who cherish us, lifted up by those who accept us. It is very easy for me to be utterly happy and fulfilled. In every moment no matter what the external tragedy or challenge, I have within me oceans of love poured into me by those who have filled my life. Every moment is a surprise and a gift. I have been blessed to be able to live my dream without ever compromising it or diminishing it. It is the rarest of things, to live your life doing everything you love. As Ed once told me, that is a freedom so unusual, but so too is the price.

In 2005 Rebecca was contacted by RTE, the Irish national television station. They wanted to make a documentary on our work in Africa. I had always opposed the idea of making a film of our work. It could easily be invasive or distressing for the sick and their families, it could easily simplify complex situations, or worse, reinforce popular stereotypes of the poor and of Africa. But I had heard of Jim Fahy. He was in broadcasting for 30 years, an award winning journalist. The rest of the team were all experienced and we felt that this would actually be a great opportunity to share a different view of Africa. The result changed ICROSS in many ways. Jim and his producer Caroline Bleahen created a powerful and beautiful film through the lens of RTE's most experienced cameraman, Mike Lee.

We got off to a slightly rocky start with me introducing the TV crew to the Kenyan team and telling them that they would have a great time. I would be in other projects but they would be well looked after. This was a slight gap in understanding with Jim explaining that I would have to go with them. I explained that the best way of getting a fresh look at Africa would be through African eyes and suggested that I might do an interview at some stage. It took a phone call from Rebecca to prompt the necessary attitude correction and I reassured the very patient crew that all would be well. This calmed things at least for a couple of hours. I unwisely shared the history of the guest house and those who had died there. Within an hour Caroline had the team in a hotel in Nairobi!

After that the only way was up. I never realised there was so much work behind making a documentary. Jim, Caroline and Mike threw themselves into the film and worked without ceasing. Jim gave me my first but not last double Jameson whiskey which is without doubt the finest whiskey in the world. I introduced them to Mary who had been working with us since the first mobile clinics, and they were enchanted by her. They filmed the gifted Elle, who froze in front of the camera, only to redeem himself when they filmed him with children. We shared many adventures, Mike hanging out of the jeep to get shots at risk of life and limb. Morten was shy and did not say much and I was proud of the amazing family we had, quietly doing wonderful things without noticing it. For the very first time one of my sculptures was filmed, Laren the Etruscan god of war. Most of the commissions are for individuals, usually a single piece of a loved one not for public consumption. The saddest was a life size bronze of a little boy who had died sitting in an arm chair watching TV. His parents remembered him as he was and in their sitting room, his eyes wide and a smile on his face. The crew filmed one of our African doctors in the bush who worked in the most hostile dry dust bowl. He had been offered many jobs including work abroad but he remained with his people on the remote plains in sight of Kilimanjaro.

For weeks Jim braved the heat and then we went to Western Kenya to film the devastating effects of

AIDS on the poor. It was an intense, demanding trip, especially for the team. Mike Lee had been in Ethiopia during the famine and in Rwanda in the aftermath of the genocide, so he was at least used to the heat and dryness, so it was harder for Caroline, who throughout had to organise the sequences, the shots and put up with me, and I was apparently 'not easy'. There were many moments throughout the film that captured the majesty and dignity of the people. We had a lot of fun, and great evenings, forming in the process friendships that have deepened.

ICROSS was moving towards an international restructuring if we were going to meet the deteriorating AIDS crisis and the emerging problems in children's health. Apart from the cyclic droughts and famines, ICROSS would need to rethink its way of raising support. Without serious growth we would not manage the growing challenges. We called in one of the most respected figures in the charity world, Owen Keenan. Owen was an old friend and he was known internationally for his integrity, experience and diplomacy. I had been invited over the years to talk at international conventions, usually on the emerging problems faced by vulnerable children in Africa.

Owen undertook an organisational review, a process that would take months to do well, and everything Owen did, he did well. Another close friend, Valerie Pierce, had been closely involved with ICROSS and she was a constant source of wisdom and insight. Val and I shared an offbeat sense of style, as well as a shared passion for France, and she remains one of the very few I can confide in. She knows all the stories not shared in these pages. Val was to play an important role in the development of ICROSS.

While I was working on some new concepts Colin Meagle was with me. He described my thinking.

'Visualise the image of a classic Rubik's cube floating in the ether of its own accord, with each of its faces containing nine little cubes rotating about its centre. As you view it, the patterns mix constantly as the colours around the sides of the closest face are turned on to other sides. Now extend this vision to three of these cubes constantly rotating around each other while each individual cube constantly shifts pattern within itself.'

He said that seeing me focus was 'to see all of these cubes suddenly shift to one single solid colour on each cube while they still rotate around each other.'

He then told me, 'By watching the patterns, after four or five seemingly random rotations, the pattern of colours becomes so complicated that it is almost impossible to figure out what the sequence of rotations was, or why they were made, and yet somehow you can always navigate back and forward throughout this circumvolving colour labyrinth to produce lucid, relevant, and inspiring thoughts, ideas and decisions.'

I don't think I've ever been compared to a Rubik's cube before but I understood this was his description of dynamic, creative thinking. It should be the way we teach children to think instead of teaching them to sort ideas into boxes and follow linear threads of relationships. Reasoning should be one of many disciplines within an epistemology. The architecture of original thought is really seeing new synergies, innovating other patterns and webs of inter-relationships and meaning.

An autotelic person understands that to make the optimum use of our life, one must enter the *flow* of life. In other words, to be in harmony with your life, to the point that your energy, attention, life force and passions are immersed in the sheer engagement of a life which is significant and fulfilling. Time seems to be effortless in its passing as life becomes a series of engaged moments, rather than the more common human experience of a meaningless drifting through life. It is this focus and concentration of energy that opens up sets of relationships and dynamics that create happiness internally.

How many people drift through their working week, counting down the daily hours of their dull, non-inspired job role, using stimuli such as copious amounts of coffee and tea, text and instant messages, and lunches with friends debating their passionless relationships until the weekend comes? Friday night then brings too much alcohol, three wrong sentences, one sexual mistake, a hangover, and one useless phone number. At least it provides something to occupy the jaded mind during the invariable calendar repeat for the following week.

Flow allows the martial artist to *be* the martial art, the dancer to *be* the dance, the lover to *be* love. The understanding is to be, not to do. That is the difference between a life lived to the full, and a role carried out while one drifts meaninglessly through time.

Morten continued to surprise me. To strangers he was a meek, shy, polite young man. Over the years he has demonstrated a passion and conviction in a quiet, unheralded resolve. He is the most Danish of Danes but a citizen of the world first. In many ways Tadju is the son I always wanted; he believes in Africa, believes in the future, and has no time for cynicism. He is too busy making a difference. His humility hides his courage and this trendy, cool dancer can fit in at the wildest of parties or the most elite gatherings. He is at much at home in a slum hovel helping a blind child as he is in a TV studio talking about global poverty. Both he does in the same way, by pouring his own gentleness into the person he is with.

One of the real guiding lights in global planning is Amitav Rath. Over he years he has become a good friend. His intellect and vision have inspired many important works on international issues. Amitav, however, captures more than the data: he is one of the thinkers who grasps the big picture. Unlike many thinkers who look from within a limited perspective, Amitav grasps the depth and wealth of other cultures. His respect and passion, gentleness and humility are rare in the world of international advisors.

I began designing three sculptures, each of which would reflect a part of my delight in life, and these would take three years to complete. They would be paid for by a commission to create a bronze statue of two heads, sisters in their thirties, both pianists. The three sculptures would be created and cast in Europe. The first and most pressing would be a life size bust of Joe Barnes, now in his nineties. I would have to capture his beauty, his dignity, his power. That would be the easiest, it would flow through him into the sculpture. The second would be an angel, which would be technically difficult to create as its wing span would be seven feet. The third would be a torso of a man in battle.

All three would be for an ambitious international exhibition called *Africa Awakes*. I decided to create an exhibition for three reasons. Many of my friends were artists and were always asking me how they could help. I began thinking . . . what do you think of when you think of Africa? Helpless starving people begging for food; hungry children fed by charities. Corruption, wars and dishonesty. Images of AIDS and disease have twisted our view of the greatest continent on Earth. We are tired of such a destructive, lost, wasted place. We either think it's sad or we think of the game parks and safaris. Neither image is worthy. Africa Awakes would share the power, epic scale, energy and fire of the ancient and new. Africa is 53 countries, 20% of the world's land, 800 million people, the oldest continent on Earth, the cradle of mankind where we took our first steps, our beginning. Through photographs, film, paintings, sculpture and multimedia, every sense will be used to share the majesty, passion and reality of an emerging Africa. Through over 200 works this exhibition will destroy the twisted stereotypes and offer a raw and compelling alternative.

The exhibition, which will take place in 2007 and will travel around the world, aims to give dignity back to Africa, to show the rest of us that this is not a hopeless continent constantly needing our help, but a proud, noble place where people just like us, with the same hopes and dreams, live and love and celebrate their very existence. This will be a fantastic exhibition, full of immense artistic talent and stunning, creative pieces, and I urge every single person to go and see it, to learn from it, and to enjoy it. Lise Hand is writing the accompanying book.

***

Dr Joe Barnes was patron of ICROSS in Ireland and Lord Nick Rea, another physician, was patron in the UK. General Lew McKenzie was patron in Canada and Dr Tom O'Riordan in the US. We lacked an international patron who would embody the fire and energy we tried to share. We needed someone who understood extreme poverty and the struggle of the outcast. I found the perfect person—Margaret of Castello. Margaret was abandoned as a child as she was a horribly deformed midget. She was blind, with severe spinal damage, and was unable to walk. She was outcast and walled up in a cell for 14 years. She lived among the unwanted lepers in a town and was refused entry into hospitals and churches. Her amazing life was full of love and healing and she cared for the rejected and unwanted. Margaret would be the perfect patron of ICROSS internationally. She demonstrated passion, courage, compassion, and despite all the odds ended up changing the world around her dramatically.

When I shared this with the various ICROSS boards I left out several details. Some directors thought such an appointment merited consensus, while others were delighted. Some recalled reading about Margaret in *Hello* magazine; one asked if I met her at an Elton John party. Everyone wanted to meet Margaret. It was only after teasing my friends a little more that I told them that Margaret of Castello was indeed the rarest and greatest of patrons; she was actually patroness of the unwanted, oppressed and neglected, patroness of the destitute and the handicapped: patroness of those in absolute poverty, and she died on 13 April 1320. Her body never decayed and lies under the altar inside a church she was not allowed to enter in her lifetime as she was deformed and grotesque.

There are very few things that really matter in a life, and they can be summarised, I think, in these things: that with everything at our disposal we try to cherish each other and make life a little better in any way we can. That we celebrate every moment as pure gift, rejoicing in its magic.

Everywhere we look there are little miracles and little wonders. There are countless examples right in front of us, of joy and goodness, but sometimes we fail to see them. A gentle word, a kindness, the laughter of a child, the gift of someone being patient. The power words and affirmations we can give, letting go of anger or refusing to be irritated. It is these little acts of goodness that can make our day. The power of acceptance and of feeling valued is so healing. In my own life the real friends are those who have walked at my side when I was lost or afraid. I never stop being surprised at just how wonderful people can be and how amazing most people really are.

I remember having my car stolen once in Dublin. I was delighted. It was a total wreck and I was not even able to lock the door anyway. I had gone to meet friends and go to the cinema. My little car was a rust bucket and no self-respecting joy rider would steal it as Dr Joe could easily overtake me on his bike. It was nearly midnight when I discovered the car gone, and I got the bus home. I reported the car stolen and went to Galway for a few days. The police called and said that the car had been found in a church car park in Donnybrook. The back seat had been full of rubbish and it was now tidy and clean, there was petrol in the usually empty tank, and the car had been washed. On the passenger seat was a pile of pictures that I used in lectures. They were pictures of our work in Africa, among them a picture of Shalos and Sempe. A scribbled note on top of the neat pile read, 'Sorry'.

Shalos was the eldest orphaned child of a poor family that has no land; she lived in a slum near Nairobi. She was 15, and for the past two years she had been a prostitute trying to get money to feed her two young brothers. She was HIV positive. Shalos had been gang raped twice, raped by a police man and an uncle. She had had a back street abortion which had caused a lot of pain. She had gonorrhoea, syphilis and when we met her, malaria. Shalos did not like selling her body. It cost less than $40 to give Shalos a course in dressmaking, and a small sewing machine. She is now working with a self-help group; she is slowly healing. She still has problems, but with a little support and respect there is a lot she can do together with new friends to change her own future. She said to me in Swahili, 'I don't want you to carry me, but if you can just hold my hand while I step up.'

Sempe was an 18 year old South African man who was held in detention because he was accused of stealing $2 from a man in a bus and was caught and beaten up. He was held in prison for three months. When he was in prison he was infected with HIV.

His family chased him away when he started to get sick, because they were afraid. Sempe had nowhere to go and in his loneliness he tried to kill himself. I cannot tell you about the humiliation, the sense of grief and loss, tides of shame that drowned Sempe, only that he was very deeply wounded in his whole sense of self-worth. There was a lot we could put right, but most of all Sempe just needed friends, not money, not clinical care, but above all, someone to care. Someone to hold his hand without hurting him, someone to accept him. Sempe is now a mechanic. He is slowly healing, slowly getting a new start, he has a group of friends. Love costs nothing. Respect and kindness cost nothing.

If you look at your life and think about where your energy comes from; it is usually from the love you have within yourself and the love that you are given. I think this is true with us all. Perhaps the journey is about discovering that love and sharing it.

Every moment brings into our world unannounced people, unexpected events, twists and turns that can never be anticipated. Some of these surprises are welcome, others are not. How we deal with all these changing situations and dynamics is simply a matter of perception and choice.

We all get days when everything seems to go wrong. Once I awoke with a blinding headache, which was rare for me. It was cold and I was in London. The heating was not working, or if it was I did not know how to use it. I tried to call a few friends but my phone had been cut off for not paying a balance of £1.28, and this would be chaotic as time was tight. I could not schedule anything in the few days I had. Later that morning I lost my tube ticket and the underground staff were very unhelpful (I find them usually great). I went to go and meet Carlo but his flight had been snowed in in Italy, so I went to meet another friend who cancelled because she had just been dumped by her boyfriend. The rest of the day continued in a similar vein until about 3pm when I stopped to reflect. I could interpret the chain of events as being part of a really bad day and there was a temptation to construct a pattern of relationships. There was another choice.

Maybe adjusting to the London weather could be fun and not having the phone was a break for a while from networking and meetings. I could get a sim card later and text people the new number; in the meantime I could enjoy myself in the book shops. We had not had a phone for the first 17 years in Africa and had managed. I had learnt to speed read when studying philosophy with the Jesuits. Speed reading is a rather misleading term as it is not really about fast reading, so much as absorbing differently rather than focusing on separate words. I realised that we have choices in most of the things we do. Most of those choices are about how we decide to interpret events and experiences. I turned a potentially dreadful day into a pleasure. As with most of our worries, mine evaporated—the heating worked, the phone was sorted out, Carlo finally turned up and my friend found pleasure in her new freedom.

It is important for us to learn to let go. The two very powerful words I learnt in life were when to say 'yes' and when to say 'no'. We need a 'yes' to explore and expand our horizons, 'yes' to learning new things, 'yes' to love, 'yes' to seeing fresh growth and new relationships, always 'yes'. In order for us to live in freedom and wonder, enjoying our lives completely, we need to grab life with both hands and rejoice in it, never giving up, always dynamically creating our own happiness and opportunities, here and now. We cannot do that if we are slaves to the judgements and opinions of others. We have to deny others access to limiting our dreams, say 'no' to people telling us what we can't do, 'no' to fear, 'no' to self-doubt, 'no' to stress, 'no' to being manipulated and 'no' to needing external approval for who we are. We need to learn when to say 'no' in a world that can drain your energies and life force. 'No' to sarcasm, 'no' to cynicism, 'no' to humour that depreciates others, 'no' to anger.

***

In July 2005, the BBC *HARDtalk* television team arrived on the plains of the African Great Rift Valley in the heart of Maasai land. In one of our remote health programmes Stephen Sackur interviewed me. It is hard talk because it is unapologetically relentless in challenging ideas, policies and realities. Before my interview I did my homework. I watched Stephen's earlier interviews on the 'net and an interview a few days before mine with Cardinal Murphy O'Connor. There is only one way to be interviewed and that is from the heart. John Hurt once gave me some very valuable advice.

'If someone is asking you questions, stop, think, and then let your heart answer.' John is not just gifted, with amazing presence, but the instrument of his voice carries such resonance and power that he has but to open his mouth and you are silenced. Stephen was tall and gracious; Morten did not speak and was a little uneasy. The cameras and the team were very impressive and Stephen had a wad of papers. He was more than well prepared and I did not know what he would ask me. I was, however, at home in the bush.

One of the many challenging questions I was asked was where was God in this sea of suffering, where was God in the injustice and grinding poverty? A good question, and one that I too have asked. He is in you now and what you are going to do or not do. He is in each of us in this moment, and in the trembling hands that reach out for help, and in the man who kneels. So too is this God in the hands of one who raises the broken off their knees and does something, anything. Whatever it is, no matter how small, do something, because in this there is God. He is in every smiling child, in every ray of hope, in every impossible dream, no matter how distant and dim.

I suppose the only thing that really matters is that in some way we each decide to take personal responsibility for each other. That we find somewhere in our hearts for everyone on this tiny planet who is in need. Our humanity is not only linked but dependent on our capacity to protect the weak and vulnerable. We will be judged by history as a society with vast resources in which over half of humanity lived in unimaginable poverty. This will be remembered as either one of the darkest times or the moment when we reached out and changed the world. I have consistently seen more compassion and action from those who have no faith than those who do. For the faithful there is solace in praying for the children who live in humiliating degradation, for those who see only themselves as the solution there is only the possibility of personal action or denial. We are living in the midst of a holocaust in which 50,000 die each day; there are no platitudes to sanitise such atrocity, no good will that gives us immunity from responsibility. Helen Keller wrote, 'We may have found a cure for most evils; but we have found no remedy for the worst of them all—the apathy of human beings.' We live in a torn world crippled with greed, apathy and cynicism. Infinitely greater than this spiral of negation is the goodness that is growing in the world.

We have a very long way to go before any sanity reaches the decision makers and those in power; they are too preoccupied with egos and short term policies to create global responses that would really end poverty. The wonderful thing is that despite the inertia of politics and the lack of vision of donors there are great changes already happening.

***

Just as God does not need religions to touch human hearts, progress does not need politicians. The winds of change have already begun sweeping out the stale, useless models of failed policies. Within 20 years global development will be so radically transformed that the wasteful agencies of today will merge into publicly accountable, efficient conduits of transparent impact. Everything will be in public view and the inept choices made behind closed doors between cliques of unqualified bureaucrats will be replaced. Decisions now made by overpaid committees in Western capitals will be made by the poor and tax payers will hold their governments responsible for where their money is placed. But that is tomorrow, and until then we need to challenge the Lords of Poverty who would use our taxes to further their sad agendas and egos. I believe passionately in the right of self determination. Like a growing number of people, I am concerned by the invasion of personal privacy instigated by a culture of fear. The invasion of personal rights and the intolerance of freedom of expression has brought a new era of stupidity and prejudice.

***

Lepesh was a young Samburu shepherd. He helped his mother look after the other children. They had often known what it meant to sleep without eating. When the rains failed they had nothing to eat. The family joined hundreds of others to look for help, and as they walked through the barren desert the hundreds grew into thousands .

Most of the young children became very sick with diarrhoeal infections. Finally Lepesh and his family found some water which was stagnant. It was a choice of letting the children become even more dehydrated, or drinking filthy water. So Lepesh and his mother let the children drink. A few days later the youngest children died. Over the next two weeks almost everybody else died. Lepesh found a small boy who was lying by the body of his mother. He picked him up and carried him. They went begging from village to village. His sandals had been stolen in the camp, and over the coming weeks he was to waste away and to become only 60 pounds in weight. His hair slowly fell out and his physique changed from that of a young athlete to a skeleton. He made the slow transition from an intelligent and attractive young man with a future, to a pitiful statistic, to barely able to speak. Hunger is a dreadful way to die. It is degrading and humiliating. People in a big car took photos of them along the roadside, then drove off. When you see them taking a photograph of you, then you are too far gone to be helped. Before Lepesh came to us he had walked for two weeks. He had to keep spitting into the boy's mouth to keep it from becoming dry and swollen. Lepesh's face had withered into that of an old man. He never knew what it was to go to school, to have nice clothes, to have a girlfriend or to watch television. He never had his own things. He knew what it was to have nowhere to go, to have no water to give his little brothers and sisters. The famine had come, and come with a vengeance. We had known many famines before but this was very serious, wiping out 95% of all the cattle and goats. Our appeals for help fell on deaf ears until the famine worsened. It is hard to interest those who have everything in those who have nothing.

***

In April 2006, when I received the Honorary Doctorate in Medicine from the National University of Ireland, I was sure that it was a mistake or just a joke, but it was to be a very personal honour for me, having spent many years in academic work. Ireland has no honours system; this was it. At the same ceremony were Martin Sheen and Louise Arbour, UN High Commissioner for Human Rights. Our group of seven was made up by Philip Treacy, John McCarthy, Bill Harris and Caroline Casey. Louise was tiny and sat by me. I met her when I put my arm around a diminutive robed girl beside me and pointed at a presidential limo with flags. 'I wonder where the big UN guy is?' I quipped. 'You have your arm around him,' she replied. She was a delight.

She was best known as a chief prosecutor for tribunals into the genocide in Rwanda and human rights abuses in Yugoslavia in the 1990s. She earned an international reputation for courage and tenacity and gained the respect of United Nations Secretary General Kofi Annan, as well as human rights groups around the world. She was appointed to the Supreme Court of Canada in 1999. In February 2004, Arbour announced she would leave the Supreme Court to become the new UN High Commissioner for Human Rights. She replaced Sergio Vieira de Mello, who was killed in the bombing of the UN headquarters in Baghdad. I asked if she was going to prosecute the United States administration for torture and the illegal detention of thousands held illegally, and for their gross abuses of human rights. She smiled and I held her large velvet hat while she went up to receive her Doctorate from the Chancellor, Garret Fitzgerald. Martin Sheen had been arrested 63 times in his campaigning against the misuse of power and wars in which so many are hurt and abused. I saw within him a kindred spirit, one who looks really amazing at 65.

The rather surreal occasion began innocently enough and continued in equal grandeur and a pageantry not typical of our people. I arrived two hours early only to meet Mum and Dad who always arrive three hours early for everything. I was not quite sure if they knew what the occasion was but they were there. We had tea and spoke about Voltaire and DNA mapping and the recent evolutions in the human genome as well as the cat's latest asthmatic developments, which were I was assured unrelated to their smoking habits or a recent attack by the gerbil which lived in the sitting room.

The robing was a wonderful affair in a sanctuary full of the great and famous. Not least among them, Dr Caroline Hussey. We both shared a passion for cats; her three were called Mischief, Magic and Mayhem. Caroline was one of the brightest, most dynamic and exciting people I ever met, with a delicious irreverence and a profound sense of culture, history and people. We immediately connected.

I have always loved dressing up. The nuns in Freshfield had made miniature vestments for me. More recently I received a stunning layered ceremonial Kimono from Nambu, a Japanese colleague who had worked with us for 16 years in Africa. This was very different. I had often worn the dress of the Samburu and Maasai but this medieval attire was fabulous. We were all in magnificent scarlet and purples, with caped hoods down our backs—pure pleasure. I am not sure how the hat makers felt making a hat for Philip Treacy, who was the world's most famous hat maker!

The ceremony began with Bill Harris, who had revolutionised science and scientific application across the United States and Europe. Caroline Casey, founder of the excellent Aisling Foundation, but a very humble woman, turned to me and wondered, as I did, what we were doing there. Next was Louise, who had sat on loads of international supreme courts, changed the way international law worked, and had prosecuted so many evil dictators. At this stage Caroline and I were ready to slip off the stage.

There is something very strange about being on stage with lots of famous people and listening to a long accolade about you. It's like being at your own funeral. Apparently I looked at the ceiling throughout my eulogy, though few get to hear one while they are still breathing. As Dr Attracta Halpin said to me, 'Just enjoy it!' It was such great fun. The reception was equally delightful and there in the midst of the hallowed walked Ronan, whose mind was something like an interstellar constellation. Dr Joe was there, the oldest and wisest, and a galaxy of friends, many of whom are in these pages. Rebecca had practically rugby tackled Martin Sheen before the procession had finished its processing. He was surrounded the whole time and was always gracious, kind and engaged. We had both known Mother Teresa and shared stories. One I loved was a vow Martin told me about. It was a special vow that the missionaries of charity take. That they will love the pure and serve them only with joy and with all their heart. Mother Teresa never believed in fund raising because she believed work was important and that money should come only from people who want to give. This is certainly my own experience: that those who have in their heart to give will give anyway and from their heart.

Rebecca was with me for an amazing dinner and I got to sit by Attracta Halpin whose son was an artist; Attracta was the Registrar of the Universities and was also beside the extraordinary Caroline Hussey. The seven of us decided we would stay in touch and Martin thought we should call ourselves modestly the Magnificent Seven. We each said a few words at the dinner; I can't remember what I said but by then I am sure that few of us could. Philip Treacy, Stefan Bartlett and I went out to celebrate. They too were pure delight. Philip's gentleness and insight was wonderful.

***

A few days later I was in Africa in a tiny school in a remote part of northern Kenya. In one class there were 45 children, all between 13 and 15. They write with twigs on their skin, as there are no books, and they sit on the dusty ground, as there are no desks. They were all totally wonderful, great dancers, very funny and loved football. In so many ways, just like kids in any school: the same hopes, dreams, ambitions. They listen to the same music on the radio and are totally awake from the first lesson. Going around the class, I found out that they averaged about a 90 minute walk to school, which is a small wooden hut with one overworked teacher who has not been paid his $30 a month for four months. The teacher sleeps in the classroom. I asked if anyone knew anything about Ireland, and one kid not only told me about it but told me all the countries of the EU and their capitals and the countries that recently joined, (which was more than I could do). I was there because most of the children are malnourished. None had eaten that day and it was very, very hot. The guys play football with a ball of plastic bags tied with string. All are barefoot. After the splendour and fabulous occasion of the conferring it was humbling to remember how much we can do together to just even out the balance a little. It's so easy to change the world.

***

Throughout 2005 there continued to be a response to the *HARDtalk* interview which was aired again at Christmas. We received thousands of e-mails and visits to our websites as well as dozens of letters and calls. Many were from people across Africa offering their own support and encouragement. Response came also from Asia, Australia, India and Borneo as well as donations from China and Peru, Israel and the Philippines. Even Iraq! One result of the interview was this book and another which will be on an alternative response to poverty. There were a few surprises too, both from the RTE and BBC films. Many people started writing to me, sharing their own journey, their own problems and challenges. Some were unemployed, others were lonely, and others were sick. Many people were very grateful for having a happy family and wondered what they could do to help, and many were struggling themselves but wanted to share their solidarity. These thoughts came from the young and the old, from e-mail and in the frail handwriting of the old in carefully scripted letters. I try to reply to them all—over 3,000 so far.

Among those who saw Stephen interview me was a man who understood me well: Stefan Olsen. We shared the same tastes in art and the same passion for history and languages. We both had classical educations and had been scholastics from the same traditions. It had been a long time since I had met a person with so many shared interests and energies. Stefan was wise and aware and was to become a source of great support.

***

Peter Homan, one of the artists taking part in the *Africa Awakes* exhibition, asked me to tell him more about the photo on the front of this book. I had not thought about it for years until that moment. That picture was taken in 1981, of a destitute starved boy called Silean. He was too weak to stand and had severe dehydration and bacillic dysentery, his urine was black and from the pain of his dying body he could not sleep. He had no water left to make tears and there was fungus growing in his mouth. His throat was infected; he had not eaten in days. I was 24, and I too was underweight. I was tired and it was a drought, and in me was such a determination that this child was not going to suffer any more. We had thousands and thousands of children to tend to, but you only start with the child suffering in front of you. Everything in me felt a sense of gratitude that I was there then to be able to change the destiny of that one child. You feel a deep humility. I was humbled at Silean's calmness and grace, his little smile and his dignity. I felt so blessed to be able to protect him, so amazed at the gift of being there. I was in a way on fire with the possibilities of what could be done. It was and remains a transforming experience that filled me.

CHAPTER TWELVE

'A single candle can set fire to the universe.'
– *Albert Shanahan*

The exposure we got from the TV programmes raised public awareness: awareness of the work we have done, the results we have achieved, and the huge task ahead of us. People from all over the world wanted to make donations and even set up branches of ICROSS in their home countries. I was delighted to see that even in Iraq, where people have it so bad right now, they were still able to find it within themselves to give to others.

In all, we raised over £1 million from the RTE documentary and £250,000 from the BBC *HARDtalk* interview, and we are still hearing from people who are just checking into our website at www.icross.ie.

Meanwhile, ICROSS continues to expand into new areas and has new targets. We are currently setting up a programme targeting AIDS orphans in South Africa, and extending all of our activities, including women's health programmes in Uganda, which aim to help a growing number of people. In 2006 we helped 360,000 with medical and long term development programmes, and this is set to reach 450,000 in 2007.

Our programme managers are all now African qualified. Morten recently finished his degree in

International Child Health and is starting his PhD, working in the areas of the most extreme poverty where we have so many vulnerable children. He works with these children, trying to find new ways to help give them a new future. But we can only do this if people help us.

The amazing thing is that nobody in ICROSS receives a salary in Europe—all money goes directly into Africa. It is important to point out too that, unlike some other charity agencies, when friends go out on to the streets to collect for us, they do it on a completely voluntary basis; not one of them gets paid a commission. Whatever they collect goes straight to where it is needed most.

In one sense, a great weakness of ICROSS is that very few people got to hear about us, or see the work we do, because we have no marketing or PR, or advertisements of any kind, so that we can keep our costs to an absolute minimum. People only hear about us through word of mouth, sharing what we are doing with others. Following on from the *HARDtalk* interview, the RTE documentary, and this book, however, I hope that we can raise awareness of the work we do, and have done, and the work that still needs to be done, the contribution that everybody needs to make. We want our message to reach every person in the world, because it is only with the full cooperation of the world that we can make this a better place to live in.

We continue to expand our medical research programmes and in 2007, with the help of the EU, our solar disinfection programme will be launched in ten new countries. We are doing a lot of great work and making a lot of progress, but we are still facing an uphill struggle and we need help.

We are in the midst of a horrendous, catastrophic famine that kills thousands every day, while fighting against water borne diseases like malaria in over 300 villages. Most tribes we work with have seen 95% of their herds destroyed by drought or famine, including all of our camels, donkeys and goats, which we would normally give to families to help support them. We need to re-stock if these people are to survive. We need help. This is not a catalogue of problems; it is a call to arms. It is within everybody to help, to give, to care about what is going on in the world, and we need people to act now.

We continue with our work because we need to. We are working in 100 villages on water treatment, storage and protection programmes, to help tribes survive the next drought. With this, we are expanding all of our other programmes, bringing our new research and findings to new areas in order to combat age old problems.

We are playing a greater role in educating Europe and the US about the rights of children and the challenges they face, to remove the myths about Africa that can only do damage. We are trying to show the world that children everywhere are the same as us, equal to us, should enjoy the same freedom and right to life as we do. We need to change the cerebral references to Africa; change the language and mythology we use when describing the continent and its people, from an alien concept to being our brothers and sisters. The art exhibition will help to do this, but we need to educate people everywhere, in every way, to teach them that Africa is a place of staggering beauty, but also of normality, where the people are just like you and me. When you think about it, we have far more in common with the tribes of Africa than we have differences.

There are many problems and many difficulties, but there are small groups now emerging like flickering candles in the darkness, wanting to do what we did when we were starting out with ICROSS, and they are now contacting us to seek advice. Groups in Canada, Budapest and Belgrade, to name but a few, are contacting us through our website and saying that they want to do what we do. I am constantly amazed by the ideas that are coming through, and by the generosity of people who want to help. Often, people in tough situations themselves are showing incredible generosity and kindness. In some instances, groups of friends are 'twinning' with villages in Africa. A vet in Lithuania, Vito Varanauska, along with a group of his friends, has started to set up the first veterinary programme for ICROSS. One group of unmarried mothers in Liverpool has twinned with a similar group in Kenya, while a group of rent boys in London has gotten together to sponsor a study of the African commercial sex trade. It is this kind of personal touch that shows that people everywhere can come together and really make a difference.

The personal touch is very important because international aid is becoming anonymous. The only public faces we see are those of the likes of Bono or Bob Geldof, and while they do highlight the problems, what we are getting is a reinforced idea of a continent that needs help from white people with big houses. What we need is to have an African face or faces as the public face of international aid; someone like Elle, who has taken care of countless AIDS orphans despite having little himself.

The agenda for the future should be to look away from the phenomenon of competing NGOs and instead start creating partnerships of equality whereby the greatest amount of assistance and support can be given through an organised cooperation. New technologies need to be used to integrate ideas and bring new programmes to fruition, and we need Africans on the Board of Directors of these organisations, because it is they who will know best how to help their own people. We don't want EU experts deciding what's best for Africa any more.

We need a public agenda that highlights the need for a fair and equal process whereby African people can become a part of the solution, without themselves being exploited. At the moment, some aid agencies are paying African workers one quarter of what unqualified European aid workers are getting, and this is entirely the wrong attitude. It is apartheid by another name. We need to lobby against the waste of aid and resources, where the majority of money raised ends up being spent on so called experts who visit an area for one week, stay in the best hotels, and then fly home to write reports on what needs to be done. At the moment, international aid is in danger of becoming a second colonisation, as bad as the US exploitation of Iraq. Africa needs to be liberated from this kind of attitude; Africans need to be allowed to make the decisions, take control of the programmes, and work towards helping themselves.

Too much emphasis is placed on academic qualifications by NGOs, but all you really need to make a difference is to be able to love, and heal through kindness. Education is important, but it won't help if we don't use the innate goodness inherent in us all. Elle is a prime example of this. He was born smiling, an amazing child, and has grown to be one of our most valued members. Like Lemoite, his touch is special. When he reaches out your anger and impatience disappear, children stop being frightened and people just melt before him. Of course, he uses this on women too, but mostly he brings a feeling of calm to any situation. He has a grace, gentleness and energy that is just a purity of heart we can all learn from. So few people have the pure joy he possesses, a delight in everything. The energy he radiates doesn't just come from him, it seems poured into him from somewhere else.

He came from a very poor background in Africa, but money means nothing to him. He finds the idea of material possessions funny because he thinks that money just gets in the way. When he visits big cities with me he looks at shop windows but doesn't see things he doesn't have; he sees things he doesn't need. His mother looks after orphans and the destitute and at any one time, Elle is surrounded by them, basking in his glow. He too looks after children with nowhere to go; the poor and abused children, and he is so healing that he makes them feel safe and whole, and wonderful, and human.

This is a natural gift within him that does not come from any sort of Western education but from his own sense of joy and his experiences growing up in a poverty stricken village.

We must see more transparency in the work being done by aid agencies. We complain about the corruption in Africa—many citing it as a reason why they don't donate any money—but what about our own nations? In short, we need to re think things. More and more people are becoming aware that the only way forward is through equality, but it won't and can't exist without respect, a respect that is not there now. Of course, some groups don't think this is necessary and shamelessly state that they only provide aid in order to further the policies of their own nation. USAID, for example, clearly outlines this idea as part of their agenda on their website. To me, this is immoral—openly and publicly exploiting a continent by pushing a US interest agenda, their policies changing with no basis in clinical evidence and research but as dictated by their government at home. These problems need to be addressed. The real experts are the people within the culture in question. We need to realise that it is they who hold the key. All we need to do is help.

The world needs to become a community, to relieve the tremendous amount of unnecessary suffering that is tearing us apart. We can all help. Every one of us, whoever we may be, has something to give. The good thing about ICROSS being such a small organisation is that it allows people to give in a private and personal way, and they can see the changes their help and support bring about. We need to see all international aid in the same way. We need to see the changes take effect, and need to see exactly where the money is going, how it is being used, the difference it makes.

***

Whenever I return to Ireland my home has been the delightful embrace of Jean and John Lowes. Their nest has become a place where those of us from Africa are always welcome. Sometimes we can feel a little removed from Europe, but whenever we are with them, there is no act; you can just be yourself. On my return, I am always bombarded with meetings, talks, lectures, and spend my time trying to inspire and convince people to help, every day, all day. Jean's house is an oasis and a space to be yourself. It is rare these days to have such a place full of genuine, open welcomes.

As ICROSS moves on and develops, so too do the people involved, and I am proud to see the passion that flows within every one of the people I have worked with and am proud to call a friend. Kevin Cronin, who has been involved with us for over 20 years, and has provided us with a lot of financial support in that time, is now working on the next big stage; the expansion required to do all the amazing things that need to be done.

Mum and Dad are on their way to Kenya to work on our garden full of tropical plants, and will revel in the veneration they will receive as older people.

Ronan travels back and forth from the Royal College of Surgeons and Kenya, guiding research and evaluation in the programmes working with vulnerable children and the testing of new and improved ways of fighting trachoma blindness. He is also working on a programme highlighting the rights of workers trapped in the commercial sex trade, and on a manifesto for the required standards and ethics within international aid and development, which has needed a serious and urgent review for quite some time.

Morten has now taken over many of my project responsibilities, including the supervision of and reporting on various programmes. Elle, Danny, and the Kenyan teams now run projects in Kenya and Tanzania, which are fully autonomous programmes, while Sally Mukwana runs the Ugandan programmes. Ed Kelly and myself continue to explore the philosophy of integration, while at the same time he continues to draw together support and help for ICROSS. Canadian novelist Tessa McWatt is writing a novel, broadly based on my spiritual and emotional journey, while Rebecca continues to spearhead new campaigns in Ireland. Meanwhile, Shane and Sheila O'Neill, with Andrew Rhuman and Paul Cosgrave, are drawing together dynamic support in ICROSS UK and Ciaran Gearty is setting up ICAN in Canada, a sister organisation, aimed at helping vulnerable children.

Patrick McDonald is soon to begin running the programmes in South Africa. Sr Mary Lavell, who spoke so well of me in the RTE documentary, is recovering from a heart attack but still miraculously has returned to Africa to work with young nurses, and is caring for another generation of children who need to be healed.

Dr Lancy Lobo is a Jesuit priest in India, and together we are working on a project to reach the untouchables and destitute of India. We've worked with him for over ten years fighting malaria in Gujarat. Lancy re-published one of my first books in India, and is one of the few who understands the magic of our shared spiritual journey.

Sharon Wilkinson, to whom this book is dedicated, has opened the door for us to embark on exciting new work, helping street children and child prostitutes in Cambodia. Carlo, with an extraordinarily gifted Chinese artist and photographer called Kai Z Feng, is organising the *Africa Awakes* exhibition. Kai has the ability to look at ancient tribes through the eyes of another ancient world. His Buddhist-like vision of another world captures the mysticism and majesty of people's souls, and this is sure to shine through in the exhibition, which will be of the highest quality and will have a deep and lasting effect on all who see it.

Tom O'Riordan travels back and forth to Africa, helping us to develop new and improved ways of infectious disease control. One of my oldest friends, Tom Bourke, who has been a great supporter over the years, is drawing together support for a maternal child health programme in Kissi, a district in central Kenya that is crippled by poverty. This will be in memory of his beloved wife Bridie, who recently passed away.

Dr Joe continues to inspire us all and fill us with his rare delight in life. I have been asked by the Royal College of Surgeons to do a sculpture of him. Tom Hogan, after 35 years in Africa, has returned to work at Spirasi.

The Board of Directors in Ireland is led by Rebecca Burrell, whose usual passion just flows into everyone. The Board is now made up of close friends; Kevin Donovan and Kevin Niall, who went to school with me; Tom Hogan, who has worked with me for 27 years; Jean Lowes; Margaret Broderick, and my close friend Valerie Pierce. They are all totally passionate, and have all been to Kenya more than once and visited the programme many times. What is important is that the ICROSS team is from every age and every generation, and this is essential. We need to mix experience and wisdom with new blood and innovative ideas if we are to meet the ever changing problems we face.

Of course, the most important people in the future of ICROSS are the people who read this book. Our future depends on how people react to what they read on these pages. The next chapter in my life and in the story of ICROSS will be determined by how they decide to help, and to change Africa. The people who read this book are actually the co-authors of what will happen next. So much depends on what you help us to do.

CHAPTER THIRTEEN

'We must be willing to get rid of the life we've planned, so as to have the life that is waiting for us.'
– *Joseph Campbell*

On a personal level, I too have developed and moved on. It has been a long and sometimes difficult journey, but it has been filled with so much joy, and I am excited about the future. I am moving forward the international plan of ICROSS and introducing the next steps—an extension of our research, sharing the message of what we know is the right thing to do, and making sure this gets through to the media. I aim to raise awareness, and will set out to give talks on changing the world while also giving international consultancy on public health and making an impact in areas of extreme poverty. We are exploring new areas of collaboration and research, always adopting new ideas and trying new innovations. Together with international research teams, we are at the cutting edge, exploring new approaches to old problems and finding low cost ways of creating real change.

My home is still the Rift Valley in Africa and I still have a traditional Maasai home in the bush. Most of my time is divided between visiting our teams in the various projects and helping other organisations to develop. I am also learning Italian, learning new methods of sculpting in bronze, which are quite experimental, while at the same time our medical research is leaning in the direction of introducing scientific and academic discipline into all of our planning.

I now have more time for personal relationships and friendships. I have more time to be still, for concentration and meditation, and for a private life. I find I have time that simply didn't exist before. I spend seven months in Africa now, and the rest in Europe and Asia, meeting old friends and making new ones. With ICROSS, I have always believed in holistic approaches and I feel the same about my own life, as regards my health, personality, sexual identity, and mental reasoning. It is important to use an integrated approach and to constantly re-examine ourselves so that we can draw meaning from the world, constantly learn, and become fuller, more rounded people. And I'm proud to say that I still have my ripped abs.

Lots of people become less curious as they get older, but part of becoming awake is to always be surprised by ourselves. We can only grow if we constantly re think ourselves and become dynamic, awake to different ways. This is at the heart of ICROSS, and at the heart of me. We have to be able to think of everything from different angles in order to constantly develop; we need to step outside of our tiny bubbles of existence to see what we are and what we can become. We have to decide how we will interpret the universe. With my newly acquired free time, I am concentrating on developing those models of integration to examine how we exist within the world around us.

We need to stop putting things in boxes, because that is not how existence works. It is the very same with international aid; the programmes are broken down into various sub-categories, but these don't exist in the same way in villages and slums.

I am taking an integrated approach to every aspect of my being; my spirituality, my art, sports, friends. yoga, physicality, to deepen and clear my mind, to grow, to explore more ways of reconstructing cognition. I want to put philosophy into people's lives so that it can affect them in a way that makes it meaningful to their lives. I want people to realise that all aspects of our lives are right in front of us to be savoured, enjoyed, experienced. We don't need an iPod, a TV, or reality TV. We have our own reality.

With my free time I am going to challenge myself and share things of significance, and in a way that is accessible to other people, to overcome challenges, to make people want to read and to get the information they read about into their lives in a meaningful way. It is a tragedy that there are whole groups of people in the world who don't read—at all. There is an incredible amount of wisdom being lost. There is so much amazing stuff out there that can enrich our lives, but it is being ignored.

I continue to give lectures and international consultation in order to raise the awareness of ICROSS and to share the discoveries and innovations we have made with others. Recently, I was invited to give the Annual Graves Lecture for the Royal Academy of Medicine, Ireland (RAMI), in Dublin, where I spoke about the impact of Irish research and work on disease patterns in Africa. I was awarded the Silver Medal, the most prestigious award given by the RAMI, in recognition of my work. I was honoured, obviously, but I still firmly believe that while we know a great deal about what works, the ones who really know, the African people who live with the fight against disease, the real experts, are not being asked. There are too many advisors sitting in comfy lecture rooms, listening to people like me to gain their insights, when they should be out there in the field working with the poorest of the poor to gain hands on experience. Only then will they truly understand what is required because only then will they have seen what it means to be too weak to stand, too sick to move.

I always feel uncomfortable being given awards because I think it is wrong to put people who do this kind of work on a pedestal. It is immoral to make people like me and NGOs do the type of work we do and then pat us on the back. The way I look at it, an award or an honorary Doctorate won't feed a single child, but I suppose, at least, it will give credibility and publicity to the campaign. But even then, we have to ask if this is the right way to see it. Why do we constantly have to demonstrate and prove that our work needs to be done? Why do NGOs have to jump through hoops to get resources? Out of necessity, our entire global operation is run on less than many executive directors give themselves as a reward for their owning a profitable company, and there is something inherently wrong with that.

Society simply doesn't value this work that we do, so when someone like me comes along we are told that we are great and doing such good work, as if helping those who need it most is somehow a concept that most people can't come to terms with. Society looks at people like me as if we are 'Holy Joes', but I am no better than anybody else because it is within every single person to help others. But where is everybody else? Where are the corporations offering to donate even a paltry percentage of their huge profits? Where are the business empires channelling millions to the poorest places on Earth? Where are the governments who are donating more to charity than they are spending on their own defence and consumption of non-essential products?

There are lots of institutions and people within governments who are doing what is needed, but we need everybody to do the same. The UK Government could do a lot more, but we have individuals like Alistair King-Smith in the British Foreign Office doing something about it. He has set up his own organisation in Uganda called Kids for Kids, where goats are donated to families in need of support.

ICROSS is not the only NGO doing it the right way—we are only part of a growing group, sharing a common agenda and vision, because it is not enough to simply be in Africa doing good work; we need to share our insights and be involved in something universal, to be excited by the prospect of a better world for all, to live a dream that should be everybody's. ICROSS was unique once, but we can easily be replicated and even bettered, and we welcome this. If everybody chose to help, to persuade their companies to help, to elect politicians who would help, there would be no need for ICROSS, just as within ICROSS there is no real need for me anymore because there are so many energetic, passionate young people ready to take over.

My own role within ICROSS is necessarily decreasing because I feel it is vital to our development that we introduce new blood and new thinking. My vision comes from this new blood: young people, children. ICROSS is not Mike Meegan, it is an organisation based around the idea that new ideas and innovations can be used to make the world a better place. The next generation of Africans, their tomorrow, is already speaking to ICROSS. I have watched the organisation grow from a small group of dedicated professionals into a multi-disciplinary team of doctors, teachers, journalists, students, healers, carers and more, and these many disciplines work through the young people coming on board.

My next book will be about trying to teach people in power the lessons we have learned. It will be a wake up call to those who should already know the truth but refuse to acknowledge it, or do anything about it. There is already a growing sense that younger generations are willing to make the necessary changes to ensure poverty becomes a thing of the past and that unnecessary suffering and disease is wiped out, but kindness has always been there. It is something that is within all of us, young and old, and every day I see evidence of it in ways that constantly amaze me.

My old school, Terenure College, is getting involved, along with other young groups, to do what they can to make a difference. That is all it takes: an effort to make a difference, and it does work. Several months ago, I was stopped in the street in London by a couple of girls who had seen me give a lecture. They were in town to do their Christmas shopping, but they handed over all their money, £200, to give to ICROSS. Another time, when I was walking down Grafton Street in Dublin, a young woman of about 19 came up to me to say hello. She had seen the documentary about me on RTE, and wanted to talk to me about it. She had been brought into town by her boyfriend because it was her birthday, and he had promised to buy her whatever she wanted. She decided that they should give all of the money to me for ICROSS.

My friend from childhood, Kevin, recently decided to replace his car and had his heart set on a Mercedes.

He asked his children what they would like, expecting a similar choice, but instead they told him to keep the car he had and send the money to ICROSS to help the children in the northern deserts.

An old woman in Dublin's Liberties, for many years an underprivileged area of the city, used to make a donation to us every week without fail, even though it sometimes meant she herself went without. I went to visit her once, and she told me that it had always been a dream of hers to visit Africa, but that she had resigned herself to the fact that it would never happen, and instead paid what little she had in order to make someone else's life fuller. I was moved by her story, and arranged a flight over to visit us in Kenya to see what her donations had meant to us, to the villagers, to everybody. She had the most wonderful time. A week after she returned to Ireland, she died, a content, fulfilled woman.

It is this amazing kindness and generosity that fills me with awe. As ICROSS has been broadcast through word of mouth, so too are the little acts of kindness and generosity, the little people doing little things that make a huge difference. People can change what is around them. They just need to cultivate a new mindset. There are so many opportunities to change the world through the acts of love and compassion that live within these people. There is good everywhere in the world, and in every person, and a desire to change the world for the better. The secret lies in tapping into this.

These acts of kindness remind me of ICROSS at the beginning. Because we were so small, we didn't have the money to be able to make mistakes. We didn't have the resources to get it wrong. Our workers were truly dedicated because we couldn't afford to pay them. They worked for free because they wanted to.

Hopefully this book and others like it will challenge people to be more humane. We need to get the common sense of older cultures back, and get our priorities straight. We live in a society of fear where we are told to buy insurance for everything from our pets to our pleasure craft, and yet billions live in poverty. We are building houses for the rich, or comfortable, but where are the houses for the poor? The real poor, not those who can only afford to spend £250,000. The way the world is going, we are going to end up with a society where the rich will die well insured in one of their many houses while the poor will already be long dead, and we will leave an empty, desolate planet.

I personally have a fantastic life, but we are on another battleground now where we need to fight ourselves, look into ourselves and make changes. We need to wake up. We all need to be surprised by joy. We need to cure the sickness in society and examine what we are doing to our younger generations and those less well off, but we are looking in the wrong direction. It is not enough to simply give some money and continue to look in the wrong direction; we all need to address the problems that will not go away until we do.

As with people seeing workers like me as 'Holy Joes', there are some people who feel that a contribution entitles them to act however they like, as if simony were still a very real proposition. A man once gave me a cheque for ICROSS, and then made an outrageously racist remark, as if he had paid for the right. We needed the money, but nobody needs to listen to that, so I gave it back and went elsewhere to find donations. We shouldn't have to owe our servitude to people just because they have given us something. We need to stand up and say what needs to be said: that it is everybody's duty to help those in need. We all need to stand up and be counted. If we don't change now, our legacy will be that the rich sat back and watched as the rest of the world died.

The joy I speak of does not come out of a feeling that all is well with the world, because it is not. The joy I speak of comes from the power to keep going and to generate the love that is necessary for us all. It is not easy, maybe not even natural, but it is another way of seeing the world and reacting to it. This is not rage spreading across the pages, nor is it a moan, or helplessness, it is a call for everybody to take the energy from my words and use it, do something about it. Everybody who reads this book is capable of doing exactly the same thing, which is help in every way we can.

This is the message I want to spread across the world now. It is where my life to date has taken me, and it is where we all have to go next.

We need to show a mutual respect which doesn't yet exist. We must help overcome corruption in all its forms. We need to base aid on what people want, and not on what we want to give, and we must get involved in something other than ourselves. We must stop thinking with a pseudo-tribalism of North and South, Irish and English, European and African, and start seeing ourselves as people, the same as everybody else. If we can do these things, we can make this a better world, and we can all share in the joy of a shared and mutual kindness.

EPILOGUE

Like all adventures, my own journey is full of surprises. Humans are made up of magic and imagining, laughter and grace, but we are mostly pure spirit. We are a curious mixture of sensations and moods, thoughts and experiences. How we interpret the drama around us depends on how we understand ourselves. Our days are full of possibilities and choices; our energies and appetites change, sometimes unpredictably. Life is not clear and does not unfold like the pages of a book.

In this book I share some of the moments that have enriched me and changed how I see the world. So much of who we are is because of the people we have known, and I have tried to share them too.

I hope that this story and these reflections touch you; they are about gentleness and hope, and finding ourselves in the celebration of each other. This book is about saying 'yes' to life, 'yes' to the inner child in us, and 'yes' to now.

It is about the miracles within us and the gift of each breath we take. No reflection on our lives ever reflects every single facet of a person. I have not written about my many frailties or little vanities, nor about some of my most private thoughts, but I have tried to share something of the awesome adventure and amazing power of life, and have tried to share something of the love that runs through us despite ourselves, and my ideas on how we can channel it.

Every waking moment is mystery and possibility. It is all choice, all miracle, all power, all gift. When I get up in the morning I am amazed at the gift of being able to see, grateful for the gift of my body, delighted with my senses and feelings, I am thankful for the freedom I have and the people who fill my life and I am astonished at the goodness that floods into my world from everywhere.

I am surprised in everything because it is so perfectly complete. There is a oneness, a wholeness and a connection, a primordial energy of life, and love, and power, that pulses through all creation. There is at the heart of all things a total, ultimate harmony, in which all things are made whole and find their centre. Within everything there is the voice of God and the presence of absolute love. It is this ultimate reality that pervades all creation and everything that we do. I am more and more thrilled and filled with pure joy at experiencing the presence of this love through everything—suffering, death, cruelty and hatred are nothing, bigotry and greed will pass away, apathy and anger will disappear, violence and hunger will be no more, and only love will pervade the universe. Only love will create endless joy inside us. This is a raw and naked truth. It pre-exists creation.

If there is something you hold in your heart from these reflections, may it be this: In all things, no matter how lost humanity may seem, in all experience, no matter how traumatic, in all your encounters, all that matters is the love you give away.

Giving should be without ego or measure. It should be from the heart and from the well of your soul. I have been surrounded by such love all my life and I am blessed. I look forward to the adventure and the vision unfolding as the reality becomes dream and the dreams of my later self become reality. I taste this unfolding and I am excited at seeing it unfold. I am delighted in the silence of my self and the discovery of all that is new.

ICROSS is evolving, and with new vision, Morten and Elle, Rebecca and Ronan create a richer future. I explore new horizons and work in dynamic teams who together search for other ways to end poverty.

Our lives are for living, our lips are for kissing, our bodies are for cherishing each other, our minds are for freeing ourselves. With our eyes open and our hearts laid bare, let us share a new adventure, taking the power of today as we celebrate the gift of here and the mystery of now. It is all a pure gift; an unfolding miracle in which, in all things, we will become in everything, everyone, surprised by joy.

International Community for the Relief of Starvation and Suffering

ORGANISATIONAL OVERVIEW

ICROSS is a small international organisation working to fight poverty and disease in the poorest parts of the world. For over 25 years we have worked with tribes in East Africa fighting disease. Health professionals work with local communities in long term development and health programmes. ICROSS works with the resources, capabilities and capacities of poor marginalised communities seeking to strengthen their capacity to improve their own health and livelihoods through the rights based approaches of participation, inclusion and community empowerment processes. ICROSS has fully documented its vast experience in disease prevention and control amongst these disadvantaged communities. This experience is informing national and international best practice on critical areas such as HIV/AIDS prevention, home based care for those infected with HIV/AIDS and succession planning for orphans and vulnerable children.

Our values include living as equals among those we work with and for, learning their languages and culture, inculcating a respect for diversity of beliefs and dedicating ourselves to long term commitment to the poor, those who are socially excluded and those who are victims of social injustice. People in the communities are empowered to take full responsibility for the changes and developments that drive the development of ICROSS. Community participation starts right from needs identification through implementation, monitoring and evaluation. Communities, families and individuals are involved in all decisions that impact, however remotely, upon their lives.

ICROSS believes that the most effective vehicle for development work is the communities' own belief systems and traditions. People have the right to choose and the right to plan their own future. Consequently, anthropological research is a key part of our work.

The ICROSS concept

ICROSS is much more than just an organisation working in Africa. ICROSS is a concept, an idea, a set of values, which is shared and advocated by a large and evolving international community. The three decades ICROSS has operated in Africa has taught us the importance of these values and in a world where political, religious and socio-economic agendas play an evermore important role in the aid industry, ICROSS has uniquely, and with instinct, refrained from giving up its values and beliefs.

The values of ICROSS derive from something as simple as caring for our brothers and sisters; assist them out of and prevent them from suffering, without an agenda other than genuinely wanting to assist. We assist them through their own people, their languages, their traditions and existing political and belief systems with a sincere admiration and respect for their cultures. By listening to the people whom we assist and developing programmes according to their needs and in their presence, rather than our wishes in an office far from their reality, the communities we serve gain a sense of ownership. This is a real ownership not a donor driven or foreign idea. The feeling of ownership is crucial in any development work; it reduces possible constraints and limitations of a International Community for the Relief of Starvation and Suffering programme and ensures success, cost effectiveness and more importantly sustainability.

ICROSS assists communities to facilitate themselves out of affliction. ICROSS has over the years scientifically shown that what we do works. Our values and evidence based approach has ensured that even as a small, bottom-up, grass root operating organisation, we have gained international respect among politicians, religious leaders, and academics around the world, who among thousands of others, make up the international community of ICROSS.

ICROSS has the poor, donors and Government represented on our Board of Directors, it is transparent and shares new ideas. This international community is the driving force behind ICROSS as an idea. The humanitarian work of ICROSS stretches far beyond our programmes in Africa. ICROSS is within anyone who genuinely wants to care and assist others with love, respect and understanding.

ICROSS as an idea is growing dynamically and with your help could reach more people.

ICROSS Mission Statement

Our aim is to reduce disease, suffering and poverty among the most disadvantaged and marginalised communities through development projects designed and implemented by the people themselves. We work through the people's languages, their belief and value systems. Using evidence based planning methodologies we aim to increase community self-reliance, reduce disease and create sustainable responses to poverty.

ICROSS is a registered charity in Kenya, Ireland, Canada and the United Kingdom, and the following offices and groups continuously support the activities in Kenya.

For more information, please visit our website on www.icross.ie/about/ and download the latest annual report, our strategic plan and five year plan.

Contact Details - ICROSS Ireland

5 Pembroke Lane,
Dublin 2,
Ireland.

General Enquiries
enquiries@icross.ie

Mariea Mullally
mariea.mullally@icross.ie

Morten Skovdal
m.skovdal@icross.ie

www.icross.ie

Charity Number 1169

***

Contact Details - ICROSS UK

25 Friars Stile Road,
Richmond, Surrey,
TW10 6NH,
England.

Phone +44 (0)20 8948 3760

Sheelagh O'Neill, Head of ICROSS UK
sheelaghoneill@icrossuk.org

www.icrossuk.com
www.icross.org.uk

Charity Number 1105400

Contact Details - ICROSS Canada

Post Office Box 3,
Saanichton BC V8M 2C3,
Canada.

Phone (001) 250-652-4137

General Enquiries
icross@icross.ca

www.icross.ca & www.icross-canada.com

Charity Number 866626385RR0001

***

Contact Details - ICROSS Kenya

P.O. Box 507-00208,
Ngong Hills – Ngong,
Kajiado, Kenya.

General Enquiries
kenyaoffice@icross.ie

www.icross-international.org

Charity Number OP/218/051/9254/180

WELCOME TO HELL

ONE MAN'S FIGHT FOR LIFE INSIDE THE BANGKOK HILTON

by Colin Martin

Written from his cell and smuggled out page by page, Colin Martin's autobiography chronicles an innocent man's struggle to survive inside one of the world's most dangerous prisons.

After being swindled out of a fortune, Martin was let down by the hopelessly corrupt Thai police. Forced to rely upon his own resources, he tracked down the man who conned him and, drawn into a fight, accidentally stabbed and killed that man's bodyguard.

Martin was arrested, denied a fair trial, convicted of murder and thrown into prison—where he remained for eight years.

Honest and often disturbing—but told with a surprising humour—Welcome to Hell is the remarkable story of how Martin was denied justice again and again.

In his extraordinary account, he describes the swindle, his arrest and vicious torture by police, the unfair trial, and the eight years of brutality and squalor he was forced to endure.

To order this book go to www.maverickhouse.com

YOU'LL NEVER WALK ALONE

A TRUE STORY ABOUT THE BANGKOK HILTON

by Debbie Singh

Debbie Singh's life fell apart when she received a letter from her brother out of the blue. He had been sentenced to ten years in Klong Prem prison, the notorious 'Bangkok Hilton', for fencing a $1000 cheque. The severity of the sentence shocked Singh, and she immediately set off to Bangkok to visit him, offer her support, and locate his Thai-born son.

Appalled by the horrendous circumstances she found him in, she started a campaign to have him transferred to an Australian jail, something never achieved before. This campaign changed her life - and that of her family - forever.

With great honesty and heart, You'll Never Walk Alone tells the story of Singh's great determination and strength in the face of adversity, the rollercoaster ride of emotions she had to face in the six year struggle to save her brother, her ongoing charity work, and the heartbreak she felt as her life was torn apart by a bitter twist in the tale.

To order this book go to www.maverickhouse.com

SURVIVOR

MEMOIRS OF A PROSTITUTE

by Martina Keogh

with Jean Harrington

Survivor is the true story of a woman who started in prostitution when she was just 8 years old. Martina Keogh progressed from a brothel on Benburb Street to sporadic bouts of prostitution in St. Stephen's Green and the Phoenix Park.

When Martina was 15 she moved to the red-light district of Dublin where she sold her body for more than 30 years. This book details the problems the prostitute encounters with the police, the pimps, the punters and the public. It horrifies the reader as it reveals the violence she suffered on the streets: the weekly rapes, beatings and attempted murders.

Survivor reveals for the first time how prostitution works; the money involved, the seediness, the glamour and the good times.

To order this book go to www.maverickhouse.com

CINDERELLA MAN

by Michael C. Delisa

Now the subject of a Major
Motion Picture starring Russell Crowe

In 1934, in the depths of the Great Depression, a failed boxer with broken hands came off the welfare rolls for one more fight to feed his wife and three children. Four bouts later, one of the bravest men ever to step into a ring was the heavyweight champion of the world, in the greatest comeback in sports history. Jim Braddock became the 'Cinderella Man,' and inspired a troubled nation.

Once he had been a contender, a top light-heavy with skill and guts, until injuries, defeats and the aftershock of the Wall Street Crash left him toiling in railway yards and on New Jersey's Hudson River docks to pay the rent.

But one man never lost faith: his manager, Joe Gould. The tiny, loquacious Jew and the tall, straight-talking Irishman made an odd but inseparable couple, and their belief in each other was unshakable, even when Braddock entered the ring a 10-1 underdog against feared champion Max Baer, who had been blamed for the deaths of two men in the ring. How the family man with a simple cause triumphed over overwhelming odds became the stuff of legend.

To order this book go to www.maverickhouse.com

IF YOU'RE NOT IN BED BY 10, COME HOME

by Martin Bengtsson

Martin Bengtsson's story contains all the ingredients of best-selling fiction – murder, intrigue, sex, royalty, and espionage. And yet it is all true.

Having started out as a bank clerk, he soon made his escape and began smuggling cigarettes for the Mafia along the Mediterranean coastline.

Among many subsequent adventures—some legal, some not so legal—he worked as a bodyguard for a Saudi Arabian prince, partied with Errol Flynn and Gracie Fields, was part of a CIA hit squad and smuggled guns for African rebels.

His story has many threads which are sewn together in a wonderful narrative impossible to replicate.

Bengtsson's voice—witty, debonair and emphatically non-conformist—sings from the pages, whether he is describing his career as a stuntman on Spaghetti Westerns, or revealing his secret life as an MI5 spy.

Looking back, he says he was never motivated by politics or patriotism. 'I can honestly say I did it for the money.'

To order this book go to www.maverickhouse.com

IN FEAR OF HER LIFE

THE TRUE STORY OF A VIOLENT MARRIAGE

by Frances Smith

with Erin McCafferty

Frances Smith lived in Fear of her life for 22 years. Married at 16 to a Dublin criminal, she endured years of relentless mental and physical torture until she found the strength to fight back. This is her courageous story told with brutal honesty and, at times, humour. It chronicles her descent to the brink of suicide and consequent rebuilding of her life.

This unique account is essential reading for all those who have ever endured cruelty at the hands of a man or another human being for that matter. It gives hope to all those who have been victimised.

One day she found the courage to change the locks, seek a divorce and let his mistress have him for keeps. It was then that she realised he meant the vows he took on his wedding day - 'Till Death do us Part...'

The names and identities of the characters in the book have been changed to protect the author who still lives in daily terror.

To order this book go to www.maverickhouse.com

SIEGE AT JADOTVILLE

THE IRISH ARMY'S FORGOTTEN BATTLE

by Declan Power

The Irish soldier has never been a stranger to fighting the enemy with the odds stacked against him. The notion of charging into adversity has been a cherished part of Ireland's military history.

In September 1961 another chapter should have been written into the annals, but it is a tale that lay shrouded in dust for years.

The men of A Company, 35th Irish Infantry Battalion, arrived in the Congo as a UN contingent to help keep the peace. For many it would be their first trip outside their native shores. Some of the troops were teenage boys, their army-issue hobnailed boots still unbroken.

A Company found themselves tasked with protecting the European population at Jadotville, a small mining town in the southern Congolese province of Katanga. It fell to them to try and protect people who later turned on them. On 13 September 1961, the bright morning air was shattered by the sound of automatic gunfire. This was to be no Srebrenica, though cut off and surrounded, the men of Jadotville held their ground and fought...

To order this book go to www.maverickhouse.com

THE IRISH BALLERINA
by Monica Loughman
with Jean Harrington

Monica Loughman's story is the enchanting tale of a 14-year-old girl leaving her family in Dublin to train in a strict Russian ballet school. She brought her dreams of becoming a professional ballerina with her. While many young ballerinas' aspirations are unfulfilled, Loughman became Ireland's success story and was the first Western European to join the distinguished Perm State Theatre of Opera and Ballet.

Not just for ballet lovers, this gripping tale also details the endurance and stamina needed to survive in post Soviet-Union Russia. Set in Perm, Russia, this book weaves a tale that belongs to the finest fiction.

It evokes the closed and foreign world of ballet with natural assurance. The Irish Ballerina is the story of a young girl's single-minded determination to succeed against the odds. It is a truly engrossing story.

To order this book go to www.maverickhouse.com

NIGHTMARE IN LAOS
by Kay Danes

Hours after her husband Kerry was kidnapped by the Communist Laos government, Kay Danes tried to flee to Thailand with her two youngest children, only to be intercepted at the border. Torn away from them and sent to an undisclosed location, it was then that the nightmare really began. Forced to endure 10 months of outrageous injustice and corruption, she and her husband fought for their freedom from behind the filth and squalor of one of Laos' secret gulags.

Battling against a corrupt regime, she came to realise that there were many worse off people held captive in Laos—people without a voice, or any hope of freedom.

Kay had to draw from the strength and spirit of those around her in order to survive this hidden hell, while the world media and Australian government tried desperately to have her and Kerry freed before it was too late and all hope was lost.

For Kay, the sorrow and pain she saw people suffer at the hands of the regime in Laos, where human rights are non-existent, will stay with her forever, and she vowed to tell the world what she has seen. This is her remarkable story.

To order this book go to www.maverickhouse.com